Bethune

Roderick Stewart

Second edition

Archon Books   *Hamden, Connecticut*   *1979*

©1973 Roderick Stewart
First published 1973 by New Press of Toronto, Ontario.
Reprinted in an unabridged edition 1979 as an Archon Book,
an imprint of THE SHOE STRING PRESS INC, Hamden, Connecticut 06514
All rights reserved
Lithoprinted in the United States of America by Cushing-Malloy
of Ann Arbor, Michigan and bound by The Short Run Bindery of Medford, New Jersey

Library of Congress Cataloging in Publication Data

Stewart, Roderick.
   Bethune.

   Bibliography: p.
   Includes index.
      1. Bethune, Norman. 2. Surgeons—Canada—Biography.
   3. Surgeons—China—Biography.
I. Title.
RD27.35.B47S73 1979   617'.092'4 [B]   78-27744
ISBN 0-208-01776-3

Contents

To my wife

Preface

Shortly after the publication of *Bethune* in October 1973, I was asked by the Canadian government to act as historical consultant on the life of Norman Bethune. Following Prime Minister Trudeau's return from a state visit to the People's Republic of China that same month, the government had decided to buy the house in which Bethune was born. Their purpose was to restore the building as a national historic site.

I readily accepted the opportunity to retrace my steps to the several countries in which I had earlier collected information on Bethune's life. I was especially eager to return to China where in the spring of 1972 I had spent six weeks interviewing Chinese who had worked with him. But I knew I had only skirted the periphery of the region in which he had performed his most significant work during the Sino-Japanese War.

Three years later, in April, 1975 I went back to China. This time I entered the remote areas of T'ang County in Hopei Province and Wu T'ai Shan in Shansi Province. I soon understood why I had been unable to visit these distant regions on my first visit. The automobile trip from the city of Taiyuan to the mountain village of Sung-yen K'ou, a distance of ninety miles, took more than five hours over some of the most rugged terrain we had ever seen. The Chinese explained to my wife and me that the area had been virtually inaccessible for years. We were only the second foreigners to enter Wu T'ai Shan since Bethune's death nearly four decades earlier.

Sung-yen K'ou is a hamlet of several hundred peasant homes clustered in a valley beneath the desolate hills that provide the inhabitants with some protection from the harsh winds gusting from the Gobi Desert to the north. Here in the summer of 1938 Bethune established his first rudimentary medical service in China, a historical event which the peasants of Sung-yen K'ou consider the most important in their community's history. In the early 1970s they began the restoration and/or reconstruction of every significant site related to the foreign doctor. They rebuilt the *Model Hospital* that had been constructed under his direction. They refurbished the modest dwelling where he had stayed during his two months there. They erected a cairn to mark the spot at which he had administered the first blood transfusion to a wounded soldier. And near the edge of the village they built a museum that records his life in line drawings and photographs.

v

We travelled east to T'ang County to see similar historic sites: more museums; houses in which he had stayed; makeshift hospitals where he had worked; even a small tunnel in a hillock that had served as his bomb shelter. On the surrounding hillsides large white stones were joined to form the Chinese characters for the expression "Learn from Bethune."

In both regions I conducted interviews with doctors and nurses whom he had trained and soldiers and civilians whom he had treated.

I returned to Canada without any new evidence to contradict my earlier findings and the judgements I had made on the man and his career. But I did learn how much I had underestimated the reverence that the Chinese people feel for him.

A little more than a year later on August 30, 1976 the Bethune Memorial Home in Gravenhurst, Ontario was officially opened by the Canadian government. The ground floor and a second floor bedroom of the house were restored to period. The remainder of the second floor was converted into a tiny museum outlining his life and career. Significantly, the most enthusiastic participants in the ceremony were the Chinese ambassador and the members of a delegation from Peking. They had been accompanied by television and radio teams to record the ceremony for their audiences back in China.

Interest in Bethune has continued to grow. One year later, in September 1977 I had published *The Mind of Norman Bethune,* an anthology of his writings and a collection of photographs both of and by him. In the same month the Canadian Broadcasting Corporation's telefilm *Bethune* was released on the Canadian national network. It was based on my 1973 publication and starred Donald Sutherland. For his outstanding performance as Bethune, Sutherland was presented with the coveted ACTRA award in 1978.

November 12, 1979 is the fortieth anniversary of Bethune's death. It is a date that will be marked by the governments of both Canada and the People's Republic of China. In life he was a stormy, colorful, frequently contradictory individual who was both loved and hated. In death that dichotomy has been maintained. It seems to be a fitting legacy that two societies so ideologically opposed to one another have chosen a common hero. Such an ironic twist will perpetuate the controversy surrounding this extraordinary man. Somehow I believe this would have delighted Norman Bethune.

R.S., *1978*

Acknowledgements

This book is based on interviews that I conducted with more than 150 persons in six countries: Canada, the United States, the People's Republic of China, England, Spain and Mexico. I also gained data through correspondence with many others in various parts of the world.

In the early stages of my investigation into the life of Bethune I gained access to the valuable information contained in the files of the film *Bethune* produced by the National Film Board of Canada. In addition to some documents, letters and taped interviews, the file included the names of many persons who had known or worked with Bethune.

I was fortunate to be aided by the American physician and medical historian, Dr. Gabriel Nadeau, whose thorough and pioneering study of Bethune's life in 1939 provided me with much basic information. Dr. Nadeau kindly offered me letters and documents that he had collected more than thirty years ago.

So many persons provided essential information that I could easily write several chapters describing the nature and quality of their contributions. Among those who were invaluable I wish to thank the following: Mrs. Janet Cornell of London, Ontario, Bethune's niece and family custodian of her uncle's documents and photographs, for helping me throughout my work; Dr. Edward Kupka of Berkeley, California, student and friend of

Bethune, for his letters, reminiscences and for many research tasks; Mr. Frank Haigh of Ottawa, Ontario, research aide extraordinaire; Miss Fredericka Martin of Cuernavaca, Mexico, currently writing a history of the American Medical Bureau in Spain, for establishing contacts in Mexico and Spain, and for her documents and translations; Professor L.L. Hanawalt, of Detroit, Michigan, historian of Wayne State University, whose research skills and generous nature combined to produce needed data on Bethune's life in Detroit; Marian Scott, of Montreal, Quebec, artist and friend of Bethune, for her perceptive insights on his character; Henning Sorensen of Vancouver, British Columbia, and Hazen Sise of Montreal, Quebec, who thoroughly described their memories of Bethune in Spain; Mrs. Jean (Ewen) Kovich of Burnaby, British Columbia, for her information concerning Bethune's first months in China; Chen Lo-min of Peking, China, my translator and guide through thirty-eight days of interviews with Chinese who worked with Bethune; and my dear friend Jim Sturgis of London whose encouragement and tolerance meant so much.

Funds that made possible the research into and the writing of this book were supplied by the following:

Physicians' Services Incorporated Foundation
The Canada Council
J.S. McLean Foundation
H.R. Jackman Foundation
President's Fund, University of Toronto
Mr. Franc R. Joubin

From 1971 until 1973 I was generously supported by a fellowship from the Physicians' Services Incorporated Foundation. Funds for extensive travel, research supplies and equipment were provided by the other granting agencies.

Among the many persons who helped me obtain research funds which made this book possible, I wish to thank the following: Professor W. Saywell, Professor D.M. Johnston, Professor K. McNaught, Professor Donald Bates, Dr. C.B. Crummey, Dr. A. Kelly, Dr. G. Andrew and Mrs. Helen Forbes.

Through the kindness of Dean Douglas Dadson of the College of Education, who offered immediate support to my initial research plans for this book, I was granted a two-year leave of absence from my teaching position on the staff of the University of Toronto Schools.

My thanks also go to Greg Whincup for his assistance with the Chinese material and to Mark Czarnecki for his expert editorial help. My final acknowledgement is to my editor, James Bacque, without whose constant encouragement, invaluable technical advice and warm friendship, this book would not have been published.

Introduction

In the fall of 1969 I was leafing through a catalogue of
the National Film Board of Canada for films on the
Canada of the 1930's to show to my history students. I
read a description of the documentary *Bethune.* The name
was vaguely familiar in connection with China. Because
there are too few films on Canadians, and because I was
curious, I decided to show it to my senior students. We
were all moved by this dramatic and colourful film, and
several students stayed after class excitedly discussing it.
When the others had left, one student, the son of a rich
doctor, awkwardly confessed that he had never considered
medicine as service to others. He felt that his father
measured the success of his medical practice by the
number of cars in his garage. The story of Bethune's life
had shown the student for the first time what was missing
from a life he had accepted as satisfactory.

I looked for more about Bethune, but his name was
not listed in any of the leading high school or university
textbooks on Canadian history. Finally I discovered a biography, *The Scalpel, The Sword* which, though interesting
and well-written, disappointed me by its lack of supportive

documentary evidence. Many questions that had intrigued me were left unanswered.

By now my curiosity was intense. I talked to a distinguished Canadian historian to find out why there was such a dearth of detailed material available to the public about Bethune. One theme recurred throughout our discussion—Bethune's politics. Before I left, it had become evident that the only answer to my question was that Bethune had been a communist, a renegade from the western world turned hero in Mao Tse-tung's China.

As I came to know more about Bethune during my three years of research for this book, several important insights became clear to me. Although his personal life had a fascination of its own, in Bethune the personal and the public lives were far more closely linked than in most people, and I saw how the scope of his life had grown with astonishing speed from the small circumference of his Ontario boyhood to an heroic role in the greatest revolution in history. I began to understand why he had never achieved the success and comfort his early life had seemed to promise, and why he had accepted hard work and danger in Canada, Spain and China. I saw how he needed to risk everything for a cause and to command in that cause. He needed to perform and be praised for great deeds, and he wanted his performances applauded.

I talked to many people who had known him in Canada, the United States, China, Spain and England. According to some, he was an unstable rebel, defiant of convention, moved only by a desire for self-glorification. To others, he was a selfless, generous and brilliant man, years ahead of his age, whose devotion to his profession was unique. Everyone remembered him vividly; everyone had stories and opinions about him, many of them contradictory. I had difficulty believing at first that they all described the same man.

Like many other families in the Canada of their time, the Bethune family believed in service to others, and their belief took an evangelical form. It was no accident that most of Bethune's associates in China, and many in Spain, were Canadians, or that he was chiefly supported in Spain by funds donated by the people of Canada through service and relief organizations. He was in the tradition of many other great men such as Lester Pearson, Frederick Banting and Sir William Osler.

The legend of Bethune is both inspiring and incomplete. This book is my attempt to understand and to portray the man as he lived.

R. S.
Toronto and
Guadalajara, Mexico
June, 1973

*You must remember my father was an evangelist
and I come of a race of men violent, unstable,
of passionate convictions and wrong-headedness,
intolerant yet with it all a vision of truth and
a drive to carry them on to it even though
it leads, as it has done in my family, to their
destruction.*

Norman Bethune to Marian Scott, 1935

A Race of Passionate Men

The main elements of character are determined by ancestry. The earliest known Bethunes were petty nobility in Normandy, some of whom settled in Scotland in the eleventh century. Their descendants moved to Canada. When Norman Bethune looked back on his ancestors, as he often did, he saw mediaeval Catholic nobility, Renaissance Calvinists, a famous Minister of Finance to the King of France and several bishops.

Norman's great-grandfather Angus, a fur trader who rose quickly to partnership in the old North West Company, was from the restless truth-seeking adventurous side of the family. His son, Dr. Norman Bethune, an artist, writer and rebel, fought the Anglican establishment in Toronto on the issue of religious qualifications for entry into Trinity College. In 1850, he and four other doctors succeeded in founding Trinity College Medical School, which admitted students without regard for their religion.

His son Malcolm Nicolson, Norman's father, was, in his youth, similar to the unruly Angus. Upon graduation from Upper Canada College he led an unsettled adventurous life and travelled around the world. While in his late twenties he met in Hawaii an evangelical English missionary,

1

Elizabeth Ann Goodwin. The instant attraction resulted not only in marriage but in Malcolm's renunciation of his former way of life and a decision to enter the clergy.

Reverend Bethune's first charge was in Gravenhurst on the edge of the Muskoka Lakes district 100 miles north of Toronto. Journalists called it "The Sawdust City" for the seventeen mills that turned out thousands of board feet of lumber from the high pine forests on the surrounding hills. Malcolm and Ann Bethune and their year-old daughter Janet Louise moved into the ten-room, frame Presbyterian manse on John Street in June, 1889. Here, on March 3, 1890, Henry Norman Bethune was born. His brother Malcolm Goodwin was born in 1892.

Reverend Bethune soon developed a reputation as a stern, determined preacher: "It was Reverend Bethune's custom to preach his morning sermon to the 'so-called Christians' and in the evening he was more evange-lical—trying to reach the young people and those not as familiar with scriptural behaviour . . . ." Short-tempered and contemptuous of "so-called Christians" who limited their religious devotion to Sunday church attendance, he criticized an elder for sleeping during one of his sermons. The sting of the attack led to his dismissal.

After three years in Gravenhurst, he and his family moved to the town of Beaverton on the shores of Lake Simcoe to take up a new charge. That lasted four years, and they moved again to Toronto, where Norman entered school. He lasted there only two years and the family was again on the move, this time to Aylmer in south-western Ontario. They returned in 1901 to Toronto, where they spent two more years before leaving for Blind River in northern Ontario. In 1904 Norman completed his first year of high school in Sault Ste. Marie, but the stay was brief.

Later that year Reverend Bethune moved to Owen Sound on the south shore of Georgian Bay. Norman finished his high school education there three years later at the age of seventeen. With the exception of the few years in Toronto, most of his youth was spent in wooded, rural areas around the Great Lakes where, like the poet Wilfred Campbell and the painter Tom Thomson, who both grew up near Owen Sound, he was inspired with a deep love of nature. He loved to swim, fish, and run on floating logs, rolling them in the water like a lumberjack. After graduation from Owen Sound Collegiate Institute he went back up north to work for a year at a lumber camp in the Algoma district.

He was curious, bright, independent and very daring. At the age of six he decided to explore Toronto. In the late afternoon his frantic parents called the police to search for him. While they were still looking, Norman walked in at dusk and explained unconcernedly that he had walked across the city, a distance of almost ten miles. A few years later he was with a group of boys skating on a frozen river when the ice gave way and one boy fell through. While the others scrambled to safety, terrified, he calmly pulled out the drowning boy and dragged him back to shore.

Before he was ten years old he was conscious of his rights as an individual and was prepared to fight for these rights. The family rented a cottage on Lake Erie during the summer months where the landlord refused to let the Bethune children play on the lawn unless Reverend Bethune paid an additional five dollars. Norman was furious both with the landlord for unjustly requesting the extra amount and with his father for not protesting.

His outspoken independent manner led to repeated clashes with his parents. Both of them, particularly his strong-willed and evangelistic mother, were determined to mould Norman into a God-fearing and obedient son. He quarrelled with his exasperated father, whom he respected much less than his mother: "Father and I had our usual hate together," he once said. Bethune also recalled that his father at one time pushed his face into the ground and made him eat dirt to teach him humility. Contemptuous of human weakness, he always remembered how his father would rage at him, then come up to his room, break down in tears and beg to be forgiven.

These strenuous attempts to discipline Norman helped form the dichotomous personality that would prove so baffling to friends and colleagues in later years. Parental restrictions sharpened his desire to explore every aspect of life, especially those declared out of bounds. At the same time the constant exhortations to maintain the Bethune tradition of service had a marked effect on the young boy. The struggle between obedience and altruism on the óne hand, and rebellion and selfish independence on the other began early and characterized his nature throughout his life. He was driven both to serve and to dominate.

In January, 1909, he took a teaching job in Edgely, Ontario, a hamlet a few miles north of Toronto. The single-room schoolhouse included students from grades one to eight, some of them only a year or two younger than their eighteen year old teacher. He was unconventional in his dress, and never looked like a teacher, but he was a stern disciplinarian. A former student recalls that he often saw "... several boys lining up at four o'clock to receive the strap from Mr. Bethune." Apparently the strap was insufficient to restrain the students, and several physical confrontations between Bethune and his pupils took place before the boys decided to seek reinforcements. But the rough life of the Algoma lumbering camp had made Norman broad-shouldered, wiry, and fast on his feet. He had learned to defend himself skilfully, and a former student recalls that "he was a good boxer. The boys brought in an older man who couldn't touch Bethune." To their dismay, Norman knocked the boys' champion to the ground several times before he fled. After this brief and decisive encounter, discipline was no longer a problem. At the end of the school term in June, 1909, Norman collected his $269.00 salary and left for the summer vacation.

During Norman's year of teaching the Bethunes moved to Harbord Street in Toronto near the campus of the University of Toronto where, in the autumn of 1909, on the strength of an honours standing in high school, he entered University College and enrolled in the Physiologi-

cal and Biochemical Science course. His academic achievement was poor during the first two years. At the end of
the first year, his highest mark was a 62 in Natural Science,
and he had to write supplemental examinations in French,
German and Latin. His second year was slightly better
although he had to pass a supplemental examination in
Scientific German before he could continue.

After two years of university life confined in the city
he was restless and eager for a change. He applied to
teach at a unique educational experiment called Frontier
College. Begun in 1899 by Reverend Alfred Fitzpatrick,
the school provided a rudimentary education, especially
training in English, for immigrants working in the lumber
camps, mines and railroads of the Canadian north.
Through agreements made by Fitzpatrick with lumber,
railway, hydro-electric and construction companies,
university students were given free accommodation. In return they worked by day and spent their evenings teaching
their fellow workers.

On October 19, 1911, Norman appeared at the offices
of the Victoria Harbour Lumber Company at Whitefish,
on the north shore of Georgian Bay, with a letter to the
foreman from Reverend Fitzpatrick that described him
as " . . . used to roughing it . . . ." During the day he worked
as an axeman, and at night he ran the reading room. In
his first report he wrote: "I have commenced work on
the road and must confess find it a little hard with the
resultant effects—blisters and fully-developed symptoms
of a kink in my vertebral column. However, I enjoy it
and am sure I shall like it immensely later on." One of
his first acts was to request copies of the Illustrated London
News, the Saturday Evening Post, a dictionary, bibles and
"a dozen, paper-covered, Alexander's Hymn books, used
by the revivalist, containing 'Where is My Wandering Boy
Tonight' and all those kinds of songs, you know, see note."
The note read "this is not a joke."

On New Year's Eve, 1911, writing Reverend Fitzpatrick
to report that " . . . at Christmas, the usual jumping took
place reducing to a great extent the classes," he also re-

quested a phonograph spring, enclosing an expert drawing and a precise verbal description of the broken part. He had never studied art but had natural talent. He told Fitzpatrick he had administered first aid to a Polish worker whose leg had been broken: " . . . a simple fracture of the tibia . . . . Will haul him to Whitefish and telegraph for ambulance to meet the train at Sudbury." After the camp broke up in the spring, Norman left on a trip through Michigan and Minnesota and ended up in Winnipeg where he took a job as a reporter on the staff of the Winnipeg *Telegram.*

News reporting and city life were still too confining. He wrote Reverend Fitzpatrick in July asking for an appointment as instructor in a railway or construction camp. His desire to " . . . get out in the open again for the next three months" was not met. No positions were available, and by October he was back at university. The year at Frontier College seemed to have steadied him. He was admitted into the second year of medicine at the University of Toronto on condition that he carry a first-year Embryology course. Free from the language courses he disliked, he did much better in the next two years, averaging 69% in 1913 and 66% in 1914.

When Great Britain declared war, Canada was automatically brought into the conflict. War fever was high throughout Ontario and recruitment centres opened soon after the outbreak of hostilities. Bethune did not hesitate. On September 8, 1914, he went to Valcartier, Quebec, to enlist in the Number Two Field Ambulance Army Medical Corps. Army records describe him as 5'10½" in height with a chest expansion of 38", blue eyes and brown hair. His health was excellent.

After some brief preparation he arrived in England aboard the S.S. Cassandra for more intensive training. A friend recalled his reckless ways: "When we joined the field ambulance . . . his escapades were sometimes the talk of the whole unit. I believe he wangled a trip to Paris just after we arrived in England and when we got our new Motor Ambulances, Norm volunteered to drive one and promptly cracked it up." He later boasted that he was the first Canadian to enter Paris during World War One. When the Military Police stopped him, he waved off their questions, explaining that as a member of an intelligence unit he was not required to reveal identification.

His unit reached France in February, 1915, where he was assigned as a stretcher-bearer to a mobile field laboratory despatched on request to treat the wounded in the trenches. On April 29, 1915, he was wounded by shrapnel that went through his left leg below the knee. Two days later he was transferred to a hospital in Cambridge, England, to convalesce for almost three months. After a week's furlough in London at the Union Jack Club, he was reposted to Shorncliffe. He remained on duty in England for three more months before being sent home and was discharged upon arrival at Quebec aboard the S.S. Scandinavian on November 3, 1915. With the exception of a notation of April 8, 1915, that read "absent from duty 4:15 to 5:15 p.m. Admonished," nothing marred his record. Proceedings on discharge described his military character as "exemplary."

When the demand for medical doctors at the front became pressing, he was requested along with others to complete his medical studies. He went back to university in Toronto determined to complete his degree in an accelerated course.* He completed fourth year in April, 1916, and, with no intervening holidays, finished fifth year in December, 1916. His average for the fourth year was 73%, his best. His final year average was 68%. One classmate recalls:

He had a reputation of being a distinct individualist and most of us felt we did not know him really well .... I would

---

*On his return to university Bethune insisted on having his name pronounced Bay-'tune, since his ancestors had come from northern France, and he had in fact been in action near the French town of Béthune in the northeast. Later, in the early 1920's, after learning that his name was frequently pronounced 'Bee-tun in the British Isles, he affected this pronunciation for a time.

class him as a good student. He always dressed well and
he always seemed to have other things on his mind besides
medicine. We used to think he had quite strong socialist
ideas and no doubt many of them were well-founded. He
was always very interested in the need of the common man.
In summing him up generally, we always felt he was a
bit of an enigma.

Another classmate remembers that "...when he came
back, Bethune was wounded. It wasn't very serious, but
he was awfully lame. He had to make sure of that. He
made himself known in this class by being a bit odd, a
bit peculiar. Everybody knew that Bethune was in the class."
In December, 1916, Norman Bethune was granted the
degree of Bachelor of Medicine at a special convocation
of the Faculty of Medicine. Frederick Banting, the discov-
erer of insulin, was his classmate.

Bethune took a holiday and saw his friends for a month
after graduation, then went to Stratford, Ontario, to replace Dr. J.A. Robertson and his son Lorne, also a doctor,
while they were on vacation. Between February and April
of 1917 Dr. Norman Bethune treated his first private patients in Stratford.

Later that spring, a young girl he did not know stopped
him on a Toronto street and asked why he was not serving
in the trenches in Europe. Before he could answer, she
had pinned the white feather of cowardice to his jacket.
Within a month he had applied to and was accepted by
the Royal Navy as a Surgeon Lieutenant in Chatham Hospital, England.

His Royal Navy record reveals his independent nature
and outspoken manner. In July, 1917, he was severely
reprimanded by a superior officer for "indiscreet remarks
made in public." No disciplinary action was taken. He saw
his first service at sea on H.M.S. Pegasus, one of the few
aircraft carriers in the Royal Navy. For the next fourteen
months Bethune remained on board this ship until he was
hospitalized for a hernia operation in late October, 1918.
He celebrated Armistice Day with his fellow patients in

hospital. Before his demobilization the Commanding Officer wrote that Bethune's ability was "above average" and
that "he has taken great interest in the general welfare
of officers and men, also in the study of medical conditions
as they affect the R.N."

Bethune always liked children. After his demobilization
on February 9, 1919, he decided to specialize in children's
diseases and began his first internship in London's famous
Hospital for Sick Children on Great Ormond Street. Later
in February he became a house surgeon and committed
himself to a training period of six months.

The war had provided the excitement and drama that
his appetite for adventure demanded but it also served
to unsettle him further. During the five years since his
enlistment he had grown to savour challenge and change.
When he entered the doors of the Hospital for Sick Children his only aim was to care for children and to continue
the quest for experience. Dr. Graham Ross, a young Canadian studying pediatrics who knew him at the time and
later in Montreal, remembers that " . . .he seemed to breeze
into the place rather like a breath of fresh air from the
sea, and one was impressed at the time by his, not aggres-
siveness, but his confidence, in his outlook on the world.
One felt that he had no worries, that the world was his
oyster . . . and that he was there to get it." To an English
doctor, although Bethune seemed " . . . a trifle bumptious
and slapdash . . . very unorthodox, even for a Canadian,"
he was also "refreshing and amusing." Dr. Ross adds:

> Everybody realized after that he was a personality. He
> rather shocked the staid young men with us . . . . He was
> pleasant though. And he worked hard. He worked very
> hard but he played very hard too. He was up in the
> town . . . . He enjoyed life. And you realized that he was
> out to get the best out of everything in life that he wanted.

While he was training at Great Ormond Street he made
friends with a wealthy Englishwoman who was attracted
to this fresh and gregarious Canadian. Her gifts of money

helped him continue his studies and maintain a flat at 14 Bedford Place in Mayfair. Even after Bethune had left London, his friend continued to send money for many years to Bethune's mother in Canada.

At the end of his internship he decided to return to Canada to visit his parents, who had not seen him for more than two years. In the autumn of 1919, the Robertson doctors in Stratford again needed a replacement and Bethune filled in for them. Ruth Patton, the nurse-receptionist for the Robertsons, remembers that he was "broke as usual, money meant nothing to him except to spend." During his two months in Stratford, she found that Bethune was a doctor "devoted to his profession. He did excellent work and was well liked by the patients . . . . [He] gave as much attention if not more to the humblest patient than he would to one perhaps more important."

As in London, he enjoyed playing as much as working. An eligible and extremely attractive young bachelor, he charmed the young women of Stratford at the same time as he demonstrated his need for attention. A companion remembers that he escorted her to a dance wearing a light blue suit, red tie and yellow shoes: "He enjoyed creating a sensation because of the unorthodox form of dress, but of course I was utterly humiliated—I was very young and these things mattered a great deal then." When the two months were up, despite his outlandish behaviour, a group of Stratford citizens offered to support him financially if he were willing to set up practice. But Bethune was not ready to settle down. Instead he accepted another offer at Ingersoll, a few miles from Stratford, where he replaced Dr. Ralph Williams. A patient recalls: "I walked in Dr. Williams' office and there sat a serious, cocky, no-nonsense doctor dressed in a beautiful hand-knit sweater, tweed trousers, argyle socks of red plaid and heavy oxfords. I can still see him with feet on desk in a relaxed position as if he didn't care."

To the quiet people of Ingersoll, Bethune was very unconventional. Always in a hurry, he drove Dr. Williams'

Model T Ford around town at top speed. He gave parties for the neighbourhood children. On one occasion he was called to attend a sick farmer and found the tearful wife more concerned about her inability to milk the cows than about her husband's condition. "Give me the pail," said Bethune, and promptly milked the cows after examining the farmer.

Following his brief stay in Ingersoll Bethune was restless again, out of work and doubtful of his future. He rejoined the forces in February, 1920, this time as Flight Lieutenant in the medical service of the fledgling Canadian air force. After one tour of duty he requested a leave of absence without pay which was granted October 23, 1920. Although his name appears in the Canadian Air Force List of January, 1922, he left Canada shortly after being granted his leave.

Back in London he became Resident Medical Officer in the West London Hospital, completed his second internship in October, 1921, and left for the Royal Infirmary, Edinburgh, to train for his fellowship in surgery. He passed the examinations in January, 1922, and was elected Fellow of the Royal College of Surgeons on February 3, 1922. From Edinburgh, he returned to the West London Hospital as Resident Surgical Officer, where he continued to study surgery. By the summer of 1923, Norman Bethune was a very successful young doctor with considerable surgical training.

During the fall of 1920 in London, Bethune met Frances Penney who charmed, infuriated, obsessed and loved him for the next twenty years. Frances was beautiful and delicate, a fastidious woman with big gorgeous eyes and long dark eyelashes. She was musical, interested in literature and she wrote and spoke French, but her many talents and endowments failed to dispel her strong feelings of inferiority. Bethune's free confidence attracted her instantly. It was so obvious that her mother complained, "Oh, my heart sank when I met him. I knew he was the kind of man that would attract Frances."

Although the attraction for both was quick and obsessive,

the courtship itself lasted three years. Bethune had no
money and Frances, the daughter of a very conservative
Scottish Edinburgh family, was cautious. Her father,
Joseph Campbell Penney, was an Accountant of the Court
of Scotland and her mother was Margaret Gourlay from
Dundee. The Penney family was well established in Edinburgh: they had money, a good house and a solid reputation. Like Bethune, Frances was hopelessly impractical with
money, and lack of it may have delayed their marriage.
Since Bethune was not willing to propose to his wealthy
English friend that she finance his marriage as well as
his medical training, they waited until 1923 when Frances
received a legacy from her uncle. They were married in
a London Registry Office on August 13. The best man
was Clifford Ellingworth, an Australian doctor and a friend
of Bethune's. Immediately after the ceremony, Bethune
turned to Frances and said, "Now I can make your life
a misery, but I'll never bore you—it's a promise." Frances
wanted to get the wedding photograph properly
developed, but Bethune wouldn't wait and she only
received "a sheet of blackness." They went to the train
with Ellingworth, who told her, "He really is fond of you,
Frances." Excited and happy with each other at first, they
left on their honeymoon with lots of time and money.
Their first stop was at Finch in the Channel Islands where
Bethune wired his parents: "Married Honeymoon Here
Very Happy Writing."

Frances was soon disillusioned. They went walking on
the island, and came to a deep ravine. There was no reason
to cross it, Frances thought, standing by the edge, but
Bethune suddenly said, "I would sooner see you dead than
funk that." She jumped across, but something died inside
her. She remembered a legend she had been told long
before about a lady who asked her knight to retrieve a
rose she had deliberately thrown into a lion's den to test
his valour. He did, but then rode away without her. Something essential in her turned away from Bethune after
he forced her to jump the ravine. He later told her, "Always
look at me through half-closed eyes."

From Finch they went on a grand continental tour, happy, quarrelling, wildly improvident, skiing in Switzerland, visiting galleries in Italy, walking hand in hand on Paris streets to the museums. Frances described the transformation in Bethune: "The impact of all this on Beth was tremendous—he was Byronic then—pseudo-romantic. And hell, did he kick while his skin was shedding." When Bethune spared a few weeks to study in Vienna early in 1924, they realized suddenly they were out of money and had barely enough to send a telegram. Bethune left Frances in the hotel room, and went alone to the station to collect the money from the return wire. On his way back he bought a small statue that he liked in an art shop. He sheepishly handed it to Frances, a few shillings in change cupped in his other hand. Incredulous and enraged, she hurled the statue at him but moments later recovered herself and quietly asked him to find some cement. Together, both laughing, they restored the statue, then went out to dinner in full evening dress.

Early in 1924, they ended their continental romp and came back to Canada. Their plans were vague. Bethune was attracted by the possibility of becoming a neurosurgeon and studied briefly at the Mayo Clinic in Rochester, Minnesota. They stayed in Stratford for a while with his sister Janet and her husband. Still attracted to the north, Bethune considered setting up practice in Rouyn, Quebec. They drove to the dusty northern mining town and stayed only a few days, long enough to convince him that it would be no place for his delicate wife. Back they went to Stratford, to investigate other possibilities.

The honeymoon was part of the distant past. Frances was becoming more anxious as Bethune seemed unable to settle down. She had come to realize he was making good the promise he had made on their wedding day.

The T.B.'s Progress

Bethune was impatient, looking for quick wealth and success. The quiet static communities of Ontario offered little
prospect for him. He turned instead to the growing aggressive city of Detroit, whose population had nearly trebled
in fourteen years. It seemed ideal for a young and ambitious doctor willing to work hard. Arriving in the late
autumn of 1924, he and Frances rented an apartment at
411 Selden Avenue close to downtown. The area, once
solidly residential, was turning commercial and thriving
like the rest of the city.

For a few months Bethune worked in an office a mile
away, but, early in 1925, to reduce mounting costs, he
combined his office and residence at 411 Selden. The high-
ceilinged second-storey apartment was soon transformed
according to his taste. In every room, including the kitchen
and the bathroom, Bethune hung oil paintings, among
them an original French Impressionist work bought during
their honeymoon.

He had applied immediately for a Michigan medical
licence and began to practise in early December. A month
later he was appointed Voluntary Assistant in the Department of Surgery in the Out-Patients' Division of

Harper Hospital. This was a vital appointment since it allowed him to bring his surgical patients to the hospital and also introduced him to other doctors from whom he could obtain patients by referral in the medical exchange market. Shortly after receiving the Harper appointment, he wrote to Dean Walter MacCraken of the Detroit College of Medicine and Surgery: "I am very keen to become associated with the medical college in the position of some teaching capacity—lecturer, instructor or demonstrator." His letter of introduction included testimonials from three prominent English doctors. Bethune's credentials and obvious willingness to accept any faculty position impressed Dean MacCraken. Unable to find a vacancy in the Department of Surgery, he offered Bethune a part-time instructorship in Prescription Writing in the Department of Pharmacology and Therapeutics. Bethune accepted at once.

From the outset, his pleasure in his teaching assignment was reflected in the students' high opinion of him. A former student and friend, Dr. Edward Kupka, remembers that at his first lecture

> ... he appeared in sport clothes, pipe and Oxford accent (he exaggerated it) and said, "This subject is a deadly bore but you must learn it and I must teach it to you." Thereupon he delivered an impassioned lecture on the practice of medicine as a modern priestly craft, with the responsibilities, the difficulties and the call to unceasing effort as a part of the profession . . . . Most of his lectures were of this unexpected type, a mixture of ethics, history, exhortation, anecdote, all delivered in a dramatic way and with humour . . . . And he did also give us the basics of prescription writing.

Another student recalls that

> ... he was a dashing, debonair type of person. He dressed immaculately, often wearing a wing collar, black tie, gloves, cane and homburg.
> He was an interesting lecturer with a dry, witty sense

of humour. He was very prompt but one morning was
about ten minutes late. His opening remark was "Gentlemen, there is no relief like that of defecation."

Bethune's unorthodox manner of teaching and his
sociability both in and out of class delighted the students.
In contrast both to the rigid discipline demanded by most
instructors and to his own earlier attitude in Edgely, he
adopted a more relaxed classroom atmosphere. He allowed
smoking and freely offered his own cigarettes. Frequently
he led a group of students to Saturday evening bull sessions
over mugs of beer in a downtown speakeasy. To many,
Bethune appeared " . . . to be a liberal (leftist) and seemed
to lean to radical causes without identifying [with] any of
them." His views must have been implicitly left-wing for
some. One former student stated that " . . . he was pushing
communism at that time and I could not swallow that line."
He demonstrated his passion for helping those less fortunate than himself, and often found part-time work for
students or lent them money. Dr. Kupka assisted him when
Bethune delivered a baby in a railway passenger car used
to house Mexican workers. The operation was difficult,
but the family had no money and Bethune refused to ask
for any. This was not an isolated case—whenever the unfortunate were in need, he never hesitated. Generosity was
an integral part of his character, but his open support
of the poor did not conflict with his desire to rise to the
top of his profession. He was a generous, handsome, highly
intelligent and charming young man, a gifted conversation-
alist, and a capable surgeon. Fully aware of these qualities
and eager to use them, he was determined to climb the
medical ladder to position and wealth.
At first he was barely able to get on the ladder. It was
months before he could attract enough patients to support
Frances and himself. In the meantime, they relied on the
dwindling remnants of Frances' legacy. Bethune wanted
money, not to possess it permanently, but to buy books,
paintings and clothes. He enjoyed good food and always
bought expensive liquor. During the few brief periods

when he was earning money he spent extravagantly, so he often tried to charge what the market could bear for his work:

> ... he not only charged large sums when he could and collected it but he took care of many of the prostitutes in the neighbourhood and they paid him well too .... He did an operation on my father for which the usual fee was $30.00 or $35.00 and after he did it and my father asked him how much he owed him, he said, "That will be $75.00." ... I said that was much more than we expected to pay and he said, "Well, make it $50.00." I said, "I just have $30.00 with me." He settled for $30.00.

Gradually his waiting room became busier as his contacts with colleagues at Harper Hospital and the Detroit College of Medicine and Surgery widened. Although he had nothing when he arrived, he was soon investing money and had bought a new car. While he was saving to buy a house, he and Frances moved in 1926 to the much more pretentious Charing Cross Apartments on fashionable Jefferson Avenue. The walls of the new residence were hung with paintings he had bought recently. He enjoyed it all, but his financial success was costly, since it further weakened an already failing marriage. Being busy meant being called out to homes or hospitals at any hour of the day or night. Frances did not like Detroit. She stayed home alone and brooded. She disliked not only Detroiters but Americans in general, whom she considered mean and common. She once described the United States as "the only country in the world to have achieved decadence without civilization." Bethune shared her feelings, at least towards Detroit: " ... how dirty this place is! Awfully squalid—terribly so. The people look ... vulgar and brutal .... I do wish they didn't, but they do."

Detroit depressed them both, and they were quarrelling over money. The carefree abandon of the lengthy honeymoon had drained much of Frances' legacy. What remained had been used by Bethune to establish his Detroit practice. His sense of the future, of his own worth, blinded him to their present situation, and he spent and lived far beyond their means. But his generosity whether to himself or to others and the ambitious scale of his life were beyond the cautious Frances. They quarrelled constantly over food, clothing and literature as well as money. She began to feel dominated by his forceful personality, and, at the same time, frightened by his financial irresponsibility. In the autumn of 1925 she left him and went to Nova Scotia to visit a girlfriend from her Edinburgh schooldays. Rather than return to Bethune she crossed the continent to spend Christmas with her brother in California.

After she had gone, Bethune immediately repented and, bitterly regretting having driven her to abandon him, he wrote, professing his love:

> First of all let me hasten to assure you that I still love, worship and adore you my dearest. I am missing you fright-fully but, paradoxically, wouldn't miss missing you for worlds. So please stay away a little longer. Of course when you do return you must bear with fortitude that accumu-lated affection of these ages.

Frances did return in 1926, but the old scenes returned with her. His loneliness during her absence and the emotional strain when she returned, compounded by his increasing work load, began to wear them both down.

He had been tiring easily for some time and decided to be examined by a colleague, Dr. J. Burns Amberson. His condition was diagnosed as "... pulmonary ... tuberculosis of moderate extent. His symptoms were mild and his general condition was good. The outlook for his recovery under sanatorium treatment was favourable." Dr. Amberson urged him to seek treatment at Trudeau Sanatorium on Saranac Lake, New York. Puzzled and angry at this interruption of his ambitious career but determined to find the best possible treatment, he stopped work on the first day of October and left Detroit. Trudeau was full so he placed his name on a waiting list there and went to Calydor Sanatorium in his birthplace, Gravenhurst. Here, under the care of Dr. Charles D. Parfitt, one of the Canadian pioneers in tubercular research and treatment, he spent two miserable, restless months. He deeply resented being forced to lie inactively in bed, and a former Calydor nurse recalls that he even "... rather resented the whole idea of treatment."

At Calydor he was concerned with more than his health. Images of Frances and his mounting indebtedness forced most other thoughts from his mind. They had separated again when he entered hospital, and she had decided to go back to her family in Edinburgh. Before she left, he wrote:

> ... my dear girl, don't worry or fuss. You can tell your people that I took your money, wasted it and left you stranded and, beyond calling you a fool for your action and I a knave for mine, what's to be said? You have done nothing wrong except to have consigned yourself and your money to a man who did not appreciate the one and was careless of the other. But let me get up, get well first and I will repay.
>
> ... you are you and a self-contained, self-sufficient entity like a well-buttressed little island that needs no connections with the external world to maintain its life and content .... I do hate your coming combat in Edinburgh—the useless explanations, sexplanations—all inexplicable with the pre-knowledge of the attending necessity (or what appeared to be necessity). This reminds me of Samuel Butler's aphorism that man is born with two illusions—one of necessity and the other of happiness. I wish I could help you. Would it do any good for me to write your mother our whole history? Our marriage has been wonderful for me. If I had to go over it again, I would still want *you* for *my* side, my darling .... Keep a stiff upper lip ... we, you and I, will beat them yet. The thought of you to fight for makes me strong.

There was one minor consolation—he was away from Detroit at last. In the same letter he wrote to Frances:

"My health insurance is $8.oo a day .... Dr. Newfield, if he can't make it go, can get someone else to go in at 411 as it is a gold mine if properly attended to, but thank god, I'm out of that shaft." This slight relief failed to prevent a growing gloominess that he revealed in a letter to Dr. Kupka:

> ... I'm ... restless at times. Too much the product of my generation to conceive my situation as tragic—there has been no tragedy since the war. I am forced to regard the situation if not with grimness then at least with a shrug of my shoulders for an entirely farcical and futile world & myself as an entirely farcical and futile figure in it. Unable to fall back on the meaningful but mysterious ways of a Hidden Purpose in life and having entirely abandoned the anthropological idea of God, there is but little comfort in the conception of a Vital Force, [and] one is reduced to the consolation of similar sufferers and one's friends become elevated to the altar like a ceborum.

His attitude was typically ambivalent. In the same letter he wrote:

> News?—Well I'm still in bed and will be perhaps for another month. It is curious how, after the initial rebellion, one acquiesces to a form of living—'I mean, *a mode,* not a *form,* of course—which is, or was up till now, repugnant to what one considered as one's temperament... Well, enough of this—I am feeling well and they tell me I am improving .... I will get well, of course, but the interval is wearying.

By early December a place was found for him at Trudeau and, after a brief stay of a few days in a sanatorium outside London, Ontario, he arrived at Trudeau on December 16, 1926.

Trudeau Sanatorium was the creation of Dr. Edward Livingstone Trudeau (1848–1915), a New York City physician of Swiss descent. Severely afflicted with pulmonary tuberculosis, he went to the Adirondack Mountains in upstate New York to spend what he believed would be his last few months hunting and fishing. The clear air and the psychological benefit of being in surroundings he loved dramatically improved his physical condition. In 1876 he brought his wife and family to live with him as he slowly regained his health. Eventually he began to practise medicine and soon decided that other tubercular patients might follow the same route to recuperation. In 1884, with funds from wealthy friends, he supervised the construction of the first cottage, the "Little Red", and laid the foundations of the Adirondack Cottage Sanitorium.

When Bethune arrived, the Trudeau Sanatorium (it was renamed in 1917) had achieved world fame. It had grown into a large institution with twenty-eight cottages, two infirmaries, library, laboratory, medical and reception pavilion, therapy workshop, nurses' home, chapel and post office. This group of buildings spread over several acres on the pine-covered slopes of Mount Pisgah, just outside the resort town of Saranac Lake. By 1926 the staff of 200 could accommodate 160 patients for the six-month treatment period to which they were limited.

Admission to Trudeau was restricted to "patients . . . who are in the first stages of pulmonary tuberculosis and free from serious complications." At a cost of $15.00 weekly for room, board and medical treatment, they could remain for six months. Sometimes a patient who wanted to remain longer and who could persuade another patient to share a room in one of the cottages was allowed to remain on the grounds as an ex-patient.

Dr. Trudeau's aim was to teach the tubercular to live with a disease that he believed could never be quite cured, only arrested. The sanatorium offered " . . . to persons in the first stages of pulmonary tuberculosis, whose resources were limited, the benefits of a change of climate amid ideal surroundings, a well regulated outdoor life, medical supervision and the most approved methods of treatment." Trudeau and his successors believed that rest was the most important method of treatment. In the period before the introduction of antibiotics, doctors were convinced that rest prevented the spread of tubercular growth. Mild exercise was permitted after the mandatory initial period of bed rest. Doctors like Hugh ("keep them in a bed a year") Kinghorn insisted on a strict routine. Even after patients had become ambulatory and were allowed the relative freedom of living in the cottages, a nightly 10 p.m. curfew was imposed by a nurse patrol.

When Bethune arrived he was immediately placed in Luddington Infirmary where he remained bed-ridden until January 14, 1927. This was the first and the last time that he adhered strictly to the sanatorium regulations. Restless and unused to any form of control over his movements, he revolted against bed-rest treatment. He had always resented authority and, as he matured, he opposed it much more boldly and openly. Inherent in his almost obsessive distrust of those who exercised power was an equally potent determination to alter and reshape institutions and individuals. At Trudeau this paradoxical characteristic manifested itself in two impulses. Whenever the opportunity arose he schemed to break the various rules that governed the conduct of patients. At the same time, he developed a grandiose plan for the creation of a Trudeau University. Bethune's dynamic presence heightened the feeling of camaraderie among the patients: stories of this eccentric and humorous Canadian doctor spread immediately in the dulled atmosphere of Trudeau.

Bethune arrived at the sanatorium carrying a silver tea service and candles which he contrived to use every day. The head nurse in the Luddington Infirmary gave orders that he was to receive his "Canadian cup of tea daily." After he was allowed to leave his bed, he put on his high hat and, tapping his cane, strutted in his pajamas through the halls. The student nurses considered him "an eccentric, funny but attractive man ... [who] liked to challenge people, to joke with them, sometimes to yell at them and always with a devilish gleam in his eye . . . ."

By the middle of January he had moved into one of the cottages with a young American physician, Dr. John B. Barnwell, who remained his closest friend and most ardent defender throughout his life. Cottage patients received three ambulatory passes monthly that allowed them to leave the grounds. Three nights were not enough for Bethune and Barnwell. They worked out a plan to evade the nightly nurse patrol. Bethune stuffed Barnwell's ski-jacket with blankets and pillows and propped the imaginary patient in the bed nearest the cottage window. Then they sneaked past the night watchman and walked down the road to Brook's Tavern or into the town of Saranac Lake. As an insurance measure, the two conspirators decided to entertain the nursing staff at a clandestine party. Under Bethune's direction a group of patients gathered pine and spruce branches and gaily decorated the cottage. Then Bethune unwrapped his big surprise: French wine he had smuggled in from Montreal. The nurses were delighted and neither Bethune nor Barnwell was ever caught leaving the grounds.

A fellow patient at Trudeau described Bethune as " . . . somewhat unconventionally dressed for that period of time, wearing a beret and using a long cigarette holder . . . he smoked cigarettes in the dining room, which was . . . forbidden." A laboratory technician who later became director of Trudeau Laboratories remembers that although " . . . Dr. Bethune broke the rules, he was not alone. He only seemed to break them more colourfully and frequently than other patients."

The devilish gleam in Bethune's eyes rarely concealed malicious intent, but frequently annoyed and even frightened the authorities at Trudeau. A small nursing school named after its patron, D. Ogden Mills, was part of the institution. Because of his background, Bethune was asked to offer a course in Anatomy to the nurses, which he did through a series of entertaining and informative lectures. On the eve of the final lecture on the subject of Reproduction, a sudden unexplained cancellation of the course was announced by the director of nursing. The subject was considered too explosive to be discussed by the outspoken and mischievous Dr. Bethune.

He loathed boredom and bores as much as he did authority and those exercising it. His mind was always working at double time. His later chief, Dr. Edward Archibald, described Bethune's mind as a "St. Catherine's wheel, always turning, always throwing off sparks and always in a different direction." Virtually everything attracted him and gained his attention, if only briefly. At Trudeau, facilities were limited for such an active person. Apart from the library and the workshop, the companionship of other patients was the only entertainment possible. Knowing that many others shared his feeling, he began to sketch his plan for a Trudeau university. He knew that many of the patients were talented people from a variety of occupations and professions who could reduce the boredom and make useful their six-month stay by offering courses in their various fields. His racing mind, which could construct rapidly on a grand and daring scale, quickly outlined the basis of the new university. To augment the faculty and to create status, he proposed affiliation with several New York State universities and McGill. No potential problem escaped his consideration. He even examined the question of movement between lectures: since exercise was virtually taboo for most patients, he proposed to install moving sidewalks and escalators. The cost factor never entered his mind.

His characteristic buoyancy and vibrant enthusiasm finally persuaded the reluctant administration to hear his detailed plans. Barnwell, who accompanied him, describes the meeting:

> He had planned it out in his mind rather than on paper. Bethune used paper rather sparsely. I doubt if he ever took time to sit down and write that out. He was, I think, somewhat discouraged by the reception. Some of the older and more important members of the staff and visiting physicians, I think, slept through it.

Bethune shrugged it off with plans for a huge party. He hired an orchestra and invited several prominent citizens of Saranac Lake as well as officials of Trudeau Sanatorium.

During the evening he made a formal presentation of a
travelling bag to the Medical Director:

> ... I don't think the Medical Director quite liked, perhaps,
> the association that Bethune was putting on the two occa-
> sions—the establishing of the university and the travelling
> of its Director. That was the kind of tongue-in-cheek thing
> that Beth could do and of which we all suspected him and
> never knew quite whether it was true or not.

Bethune's clever stunts and his apparent enjoyment of
life at Trudeau masked his growing concern for his marriage, his health and his future as a medical practitioner.
During the first few weeks at Trudeau he had tried unsuc-
cessfully to find a doctor to substitute for him in Detroit.
Since he was reluctant to return there, he sold the practice
to a young Detroit physician, Dr. Joseph Wruble. The purchase price of $5,000 included furniture, books and
instruments. Bethune's first and only private practice had
ended.

But money brought him back to "awfully squalid" Detroit. After he left Trudeau, he returned to his teaching
duties near the end of March, 1927. He wrote to Ruth
Patton: "I simply hate it. The city tires me out and I am
exhausted. I am not fit to be up yet but it was necessary
to come back." The question of money related directly
to Frances. A few weeks before he learned that he had
tuberculosis, he had fortunately taken out an insurance
policy that included a monthly disability benefit. From
February, 1927, to January, 1934, he received a monthly
income of $150.00 and from this sum he attempted to
pay his expenses at Trudeau, his debts and to send something to Frances, but it was not enough.

After six months' separation and with his world caving
in, his need for her was growing. He begged her to return:

> Do you remember the nice room with its ... parapets of
> books?—Oh you must & not all your memories are bitter,
> are they dear? ... I know you don't want me to love you

but I do. I don't care what you say or do to me—I love
you more than I ever have.... Now I want to see you.
Now I think I can talk with you and understand you and
you me...

His repeated entreaties failed to move Frances. She felt
forced to take a stand against him and, in June, 1927,
she initiated divorce proceedings in Detroit.

Meanwhile Bethune's physical condition worsened and
in the early summer he returned to Trudeau, prepared
to accept both bed rest and the divorce as inevitable. The
darker side of his nature became more obvious; super-
ficially the frivolous prankster, to friends he was obviously
despondent: "... Bethune felt that we were under sen-
tence here..., that we were all outliving our days
and ... following merely a dance of death. There was no
hope for any of us." He was on the verge of losing hope
entirely, having almost convinced himself that escape from
tuberculosis was impossible. He repeatedly described to
Barnwell his version of the perfect method of committing
suicide, a combination of morphine and drowning.

His depression suddenly turned to fury when he received
a message from Frances describing how she had been mal-
treated by a friend she had been seeing since the separation.
His fury mounted as he thought about her, and he decided
impulsively to kill the man. Physically weak and almost
penniless, he left Trudeau and went to Pittsburgh where
Frances' friend, a wealthy businessman, was staying.
Bethune bought a pistol and registered in a hotel. He telephoned the man, using an assumed name, and invited
him to his room for a drink. He planned to call the police
after shooting him and surrender himself. When the man
arrived, Bethune confronted him with the pistol, revealed
his identity, and said he was going to kill him. To Bethune's
surprise, the man stood immobile in the centre of the room.
Bethune demanded that he defend himself. Standing limp-
ly, his hands at his sides, the man replied in a low voice,
"Go ahead. Shoot. I guess I deserve it anyway." Taken
aback by the man's unexpected reaction, Bethune hesi-

tated, then struck the man several times on the face with the pistol. The man staggered, but still made no attempt to fight back. Blood was streaming from the cuts on his head.

The sight of the man's bloodied face shocked Bethune into a realization of what he was doing. He also felt pity for the man who, by not resisting, was apparently admitting his guilt. Bethune threw the gun on the bed and helped the man to a chair. After treating his wounds, he brought out a bottle of liquor which they drank together. Later, when it was dark, he turned up the man's coat collar to conceal his face, helped him into the elevator and onto the street where he sent him to his hotel in a taxi. That night, Bethune took the train back to Saranac Lake.*

This bizarre incident ended his growing self-pity and feelings of futility. His medical training and his instincts denied him the luxury of vengeance by murder or suicide by despair, and he resolved to make a determined effort to cure his own sickness. Completely out of patience with the medical treatment that had produced no change in his condition, he studied books on tuberculosis in the Trudeau Library and decided that his condition might be improved through the application of a treatment known as artificial pneumothorax. A hollow needle was inserted between the ribs through which air was pumped into the chest cavity but outside the lung. The air pressure collapsed the lung and allowed it to rest. Provided that the lung or that part which was diseased ceased to function, the spread of the tuberculosis could be arrested and the infected area given a chance to heal.

Pneumothorax was a known form of treatment at Trudeau: Dr. Trudeau himself had credited this technique with having prolonged his life for several years. On the other hand, the conservative medical practitioners were

---

*Bethune brought back a bloody towel from the hotel which he showed to one of his friends at Trudeau as he described the incident. Several years later in a conversation with his friend, Louis Huot, he told this story explaining how obsessed he had been by Frances and how little he had valued his chances of surviving tuberculosis in 1927.

reluctant to resort to pneumothorax, preferring simple bed rest. As soon as Bethune discovered this form of treatment he badgered the medical staff for an operation. At last, after repeated refusals, the exasperated doctors invited him to explain why he believed his case required artificial pneumothorax. Before his medical staff and Bethune, Dr. Lawrason Brown carefully described the inherent risks in this kind of treatment, including the possibility of puncturing the lung. Brown had hardly finished speaking when Bethune rose, and, melodramatically baring his chest, announced "Gentlemen, I welcome the risk!" His theatrics and persistence finally persuaded the hesitant physicians. After an x-ray of his chest supported Bethune's self-diagnosis, Dr. Earl Leroy Warren, a resident physician, was chosen by Bethune to administer the artificial pneumothorax.

On the same day Bethune learned that the Michigan court had issued the final divorce decree. Already almost hopelessly in debt, Bethune was ordered to pay Frances $1,500.00 in cash and $25,000.00 at the rate of $100.00 monthly. He read the telegram, handed it to John Barnwell, then wired Frances his congratulations and a proposal of marriage. Bethune always valued and respected Frances throughout the many crises of their relationship, and he knew that the worst problems between them were caused by his own dominating nature. He had probably resolved to wipe out this failure and to regain his pride and his love with one last desperate effort.

Three days later, on the morning of October 27, 1927, Dr. Warren gave Bethune the pneumothorax treatment. An hour after the operation, Dr. Warren visited him in the Lea Cottage. He recalls Bethune's condition:

... he was in good condition but was complaining of dyspnea [shortness of breath] ... I finally persuaded him to go to the x-ray department for a fluoroscopy. The fluoroscopy revealed 65% collapse of the lung. I could not persuade him to enter the infirmary or to accept transportation to his cottage which was about 100 yards from the x-ray department and was partially uphill.

Deeply conscious of his self-image, Bethune chose to endure the extreme fatigue of walking up the hill with only one lung functioning properly.

When Dr. Warren returned to check on him, he found Bethune standing on a chair placed on a table, a paint brush in his hand. Around the walls of the Lea Cottage was a five-foot high sheet of wrapping paper Bethune had found in the laundry room. Between coughs he was bending to dip his brush into various paints that littered the table. The mural eventually covered almost sixty feet of paper. For several days he worked feverishly to complete what he called "The T.B.'s Progress." Ranged in a series of nine panels was an allegorical dramatization of his life and death. Beneath each panel was a descriptive verse. The drawings show Bethune pursued from birth by the tubercle bacillus, represented by a pterodactyl. Undaunted by this perpetually hovering menace, he is full of confidence and enters his early manhood on a Spanish galleon named "Youth at the Helm." Soon he is attracted by the Sirens of Fame, Success and Wealth who inhabit the "Castle of Heart's Desire," high on a rocky promontory. Just as he prepares to enter the castle, he is savagely attacked by a swarm of t.b. bats. Down he plummets to a rocky abyss through which flows a red river representing haemorrhage. During his fall he is horrified to discover that the castle is merely a "Hollywood set."

Lying almost hopelessly diseased at the bottom of the chasm he discovers another castle, this one representing Trudeau Sanatorium. After slowly making his way to the sanatorium, he gains temporary shelter from the marauding bats. But he has not learned his lesson and the Siren of Spurious Fame seductively lures him from the sanctuary back to the city where he again falls prey to the winged creatures of disease. Summoning his remaining strength and "with a small sputum cup strapped to his cadaverous body," he attempts to reach Arizona. He fails. On the way he is overtaken by the "kind Angel of Death." In the final panel, he is lying in the arms of the Angel of Death who stands above a graveyard where Bethune and six fellow patients are buried.

The emotional outpourings in "The T.B.'s Progress" show Bethune in a furious despair. Each of the seven men in the Lea Cottage had been asked by Bethune to choose his date of death, and he recorded these on the tombstones. He chose his own as 1932. The prediction of an early death was not surprising. A patient whose bed was next to Bethune's was often wakened in the middle of the night by his coughing which was so severe he was certain Bethune would not last until morning. In 1932 Bethune wrote: "How wrong I was, in the face of what has happened since, is really laughable to look back on."

In a few weeks his lung seemed to be responding well to the pneumothorax and his doctors agreed to release him on December 10, 1927. After he left Trudeau he continued to receive pneumothorax refills around his left lung for several years but his general condition had improved remarkably since his arrival a year before. He had gained fifteen pounds and, despite the retention of the pneumothorax treatment, he could walk an unlimited distance without loss of breath.*

The effect of the Trudeau experience upon Bethune was profound. For the first time in his life he became

*One of the several legends concerning Bethune is that the pneumothorax treatment saved him from an imminent death. There is no clinical evidence of this, and, although Bethune himself became an aggressive advocate of collapse therapy because of its very rapid beneficial action in his own case, it is much more likely that it accelerated his recovery rather than saved him from certain death. His pulmonary tuberculosis was moderately advanced on his admission and his general chances of having the disease arrested were favourable. Upon discharge his range of pulse, which had been 62-88, had risen to 76-116. His temperature, 98.2° on admission, was 97.8° on discharge. His sputum had been converted from positive to negative. His weight, 161¾ on admission, had risen to 176½, eight pounds above the standard. He left with the disease stabilized in his left lung.

deeply introspective. In a description of the effect of sanatorium life on the tubercular patient he wrote:

> In the sanatorium, perhaps for the first time, he has the
> opportunity to think. Contemplation becomes a substitution
> for action. The result is a deepening of his intellectual and
> spiritual life.
>
> Realities change their nature—the unimportant becomes
> the important and the formerly essential becomes the super-
> fluous. It is only the dull and unimaginative who can lie
> in bed in a sanatorium for six months or a year and fail
> to rise a better and finer person. Life should be enriched
> and not impoverished by this retreat from the world.

Until he was stricken with tuberculosis he had been under
the spell of the Sirens of Fame, Success and Wealth. After
Trudeau he renounced his quest for wealth and rein-
terpreted his conception of Fame and Success. One of the
inhabitants of the Lea Cottage overheard Bethune explaining that his attitude to life had changed and that he
planned " . . . to find something I can do for the human
race, something great, and I am going to do it before
I die." He frequently spoke of his destiny and of a sense
of duty stemming from his parents' strictures which
appeared to him as part of that destiny. In the first panel
of his mural, the Angel of Fate unrolls a scroll which reveals
his future. In his description Bethune notes that " . . . this
theory of predestination is probably a relic of my Scotch
ancestors." The sense of commitment present since his
youth had surfaced only irregularly, but it was about to
assume a shape that would direct him in the future.

Bethune was determined to become a thoracic surgeon
and cure tuberculosis victims. There was a religious aspect
to this commitment. Bethune, a modern Loyola, had been
saved by the intervention, not of God, but of science and
his own inflexible will. There was also an element of the
highly dramatic in the decision. Chest surgery was a relatively unexplored area, and the moment was right to cross
this new frontier of medicine.

Luck favoured Bethune. Near Saranac Lake at Montreal's Royal Victoria Hospital was the Canadian pioneer in thoracic surgery, Dr. Edward Archibald. Archibald frequently sent patients to Trudeau and was regularly consulted by the staff physicians there. Bethune wrote Archibald requesting an opportunity to train under him, and Archibald agreed to accept Bethune if he were willing to obtain some basic training in biochemistry at the New York State Hospital for Incipient Tuberculosis at Ray Brook, New York, five miles from Saranac Lake.

In January, 1928, Bethune went to the Ray Brook Hospital, where the Medical Director, a fellow Canadian, Dr. Harry Bray, gave him a room and placed him on the payroll at a salary of $100.00 per month. Bethune "... arrived with fancy English baggage, including a leather hat box ... his moustache waxed, and full of energy and original ideas. He kept the sanatorium in a ferment." During the day he worked with the Director of the Laboratory, Dr. David T. Smith and Dr. Julius Lane Wilson. In the evenings he skied over Mt. Baker to visit his friends at Trudeau and returned at midnight.

He spent three months at Ray Brook where he "... learned more about bacteriology ... than most graduate students learn in three years." Smith and Wilson had earlier abandoned a research project which Bethune's enthusiasm now inspired them to resume. Under their experienced guidance, Bethune reassembled the data and completed the project on the study of pseudo-tuberculosis in rats. The findings were later published. Almost two years earlier he had written to Edward Kupka: "I think it is a good thing to do some lab work. It reduces theories in such a devastating fashion. Most of our imaginative men in medicine are laboratory workers."

In April, 1928, Bethune left Ray Brook for Montreal to begin his work with Dr. Archibald. At the age of thirty-eight, when most doctors are beginning to enjoy an established practice, a home, family and good income, Bethune was broke, divorced and beginning a new career.

Second Chances

Tuberculosis was identified by the Babylonians, Greeks and Hindus, who noted its symptoms and recorded its disastrous effects but lacked the medical knowledge to cure it. Not until the nineteenth century did science advance significantly towards a cure. In the same century, during the Romantic Age, it acquired a fashionable notoriety. Alexander Dumas père, whose son wrote *La Dame aux Camélias* in which the heroine is a beautiful consumptive, wrote: "In 1823 and 1824, it was the fashion to suffer from the lungs; everybody was consumptive, poets especially; it was good form to spit blood after each emotion that was at all sensational and to die before reaching the age of thirty." Many artists in all fields did suffer and die from tuberculosis, among them writers such as Keats, Stevenson, Elizabeth Barrett Browning and Goethe, composers (Chopin), and painters (Gauguin and Modigliani). Although science could prove no connection, their deaths led to a common belief that genius and tuberculosis and even diseases in general were inextricably linked. Mrs. Browning once overheard a patient ask her doctor, "Is it possible that genius is only scrofula?"

Bethune was aware of the mythology of the "white

plague" and his romantic nature was strongly influenced by it. A friend who discussed tuberculosis with Bethune remembers that "He kept saying, '. . . tuberculosis has an effect on the brain. It makes you think faster. You become more aware of things' . . . he seemed absolutely convinced of this and also the fact [that] t.b. had developed . . . his sensitivity and his artistic sense." His two favourite authors were Katherine Mansfield and D.H. Lawrence, both victims of tuberculosis. However, his romantic nature did not impair his scientific interest in the disease, which he knew remained a challenge to medical science.

When he arrived in Montreal, the mortality rate of tuberculosis in the Province of Quebec was the highest in the Dominion of Canada. Only four other causes of death ranked ahead of tuberculosis, from which almost 3,000 Quebecois died in 1925. More than 800 of these were from Montreal. Perhaps no one was more aware of its deadly nature than Archibald, who in 1928 was appointed Chief Surgeon of Montreal's Royal Victoria Hospital. He was also Professor of Surgery and Chairman of McGill University's Surgical Department. The Royal Victoria appointment gave him the opportunity to begin the experimental work in thoracic surgery that he had longed to do and, aided by a number of grants, he established the Medico-Pulmonary Surgical Clinic. He chose Norman Bethune as his First Assistant.

Bethune was assigned a dual role. When he was not observing or assisting Archibald in the operating room, learning the techniques of thoracic surgery, he was free to direct research projects of his choice in the laboratory. The work appealed to Bethune and he liked Archibald who, he told Frances, was "the outstanding figure in chest surgery in America and a most charming fellow." Within a year he had started a series of investigations, completed several, and published four articles. During the next four years at the Clinic he wrote or gathered data for ten scientific papers which he read at national and international medical conferences. All of them were concise, timely and based on sound and inventive research.

He frequently experimented on himself to prove his unconventional theories. For example, he believed that blood from pulmonary haemorrhages was soon absorbed by the body although the x-ray technicians disagreed, stating that radiographs of patients with such haemorrhages indicated miliary tuberculosis. To test his theory Bethune had a rubber catheter inserted down his windpipe and, while he slept, an intern introduced blood into one of his lungs through the catheter. The following morning an x-ray showed that the blood had been absorbed as he had predicted.

His most significant research led to the invention of a variety of surgical instruments. Often when he was operating he became dissatisfied with an instrument and hurled it to the floor in anger. Later he worked on its design until he had either improved or replaced the instrument. The underlying motive for this marked creative ability was revealed in an article in which he described several of his inventions. Referring in general to the inventor of surgical instruments he wrote, "His dissatisfaction with the old, impatience with slowness and inefficiency, are characteristics of his age. Even variation for its own sake, as an artistic gesture of freedom from conventional design, is quite in the modern manner."

His success was rapid. The 1932 catalogue of medical supplies published by Pilling and Company of Philadelphia featured a full page of Bethune's instruments. Dr. Barnwell remarked: "On our visits to the Royal Victoria you literally stumbled over discarded instruments which Bethune had designed but became impatient with and designed anew." Most widely used was his pneumothorax apparatus. Almost equally popular were his rib shears, which, like the pneumothorax apparatus, were not an original design. Bethune was struck one day in a shoe repair store by the possibility of adapting leather-cutting shears for surgical purposes. He blunted the points on a pair of shears, placed rubber grips on the handles, ordered stiffer steel and used them with great success in surgery. A former student commented on his creative ability: "He was fantastic in the amount of things he produced in the way of surgical instruments. The pneumothorax machine that we used throughout Victoria for the next 20 years . . . was his, a beautiful compact piece of equipment that I used many times. He had a rib spreader. He originated what we called the Iron Houseman. He had his own rib shears."

During the 1930's, the pioneering period of thoracic surgery, his instruments were highly regarded by thoracic surgeons in Canada, England and the United States. With the introduction of chemotherapeutic treatment in the late 1940's, collapse therapy declined rapidly and the pneumothorax apparatus went into disuse. Of his inventions only the Bethune Rib Shears remain in use today. As he once wrote, "The whole backward path of surgery is littered, like the plains of the American desert, with the out-worn and clumsy relics of technical advances."

His research, writing and inventions were valued by his chief and colleagues. Archibald later wrote:

> . . . he did a great deal for the clinic. He kept it together, devoted his whole time to it, was enthusiastic, invented instruments, and did generally satisfactory work . . . . I recognized his ability and was sincerely grateful for the reputation of the hospital and thereby for myself.

Shortly after his arrival Bethune was awarded a research grant by P.P. Cowans, Archibald's stockbroker and personal friend. He wrote to Frances: "I told Archibald a couple of months ago I would be forced to leave as I couldn't live on my income. He was keen that I should stay and offered me this fellowship at $1500 a year." His intensity, inventiveness and enthusiasm soon labelled him as a man who "had flash ideas that would come a mile a minute." When he was at the hospital, there was little time for small talk. At the dinner hour in the lunch room he tested his theories on his colleagues using the wallpaper to sketch diagrams as ideas cascaded from his mind. Long after most doctors had left the hospital, Bethune remained to finish his experiments.

So complete was his absorption in his work that he some-times missed meetings, broke promises, and was late for operations. He once persuaded a fellow researcher to allow him to dissect an expensive cadaver his department had just purchased by promising to restrict his investigations to the chest area. Bethune began to work. When the col-league returned several hours later, he was astonished to find that in his fascination Bethune had dissected the entire body.

His surgical training and experimental work brought him into contact with McGill medical students in training at the Royal Victoria Hospital. This contact was increased after 1931 when he and Archibald taught a course, "Diag-nosis and Surgical Treatment of Pulmonary and Pleural Diseases." His teaching style was the same as in Detroit, much more personal and less formal than other instructors. According to one former student, he was also more impres-sive:

> Bethune would come in in a jaunty way and jump up on a stretcher, his legs swinging and would ask, "What's new in our world?" and then he would ask us what we wanted to talk about.... Bethune was perhaps more dramatic and stimulating than some of the men who had the job of teach-ing us formerly.

He tried to teach the same kind of probing thorough scrutiny of every theory and every problem that he himself practised. Another former student recalls Bethune's teach-ing methods:

> He hated obscure ... baseless arguments .... That was the kind of thing we liked because ... students in our day were inclined to accept things unquestioningly. They were ex-pected to vomit these things out on the examination paper. As a student, if you disagreed with Bethune, he welcomed that. This was very valuable to him. He was a breath of pungent air, but it was good. We would argue with him and question him. He was a good teacher, stimulating. His breezy manner and his iconoclasm shocked some students.

He was scathing about doctors who relied on auscultation to determine physical signs of pulmonary tuberculosis. He called them "the fellows with the stethoscopes" and, holding a stethoscope aloft among a group of students, he would admonish them, "If you are called to see a chest case, leave this at home." Bethune, the modernist, believed that x-rays were more efficient and reliable.

He was invited to address a medical fraternity in 1929. A student receiving the initiation rites remembers his speech:

> The self-assured looks of my future fraternity brothers, all upper classmen, [changed because] when Dr. Bethune began to speak he didn't congratulate us on our wisdom of choosing Phi Rho Sigma as a Fraternity, Montreal as the city, McGill as an alma mater, medicine as the profession but shocked those awaiting imminent beatification, i.e., some of the final year medics, by stating bluntly, "Success is a whore. She will lead you on and on, then drop you.... More joy and satisfaction exists in the youth with 50¢ in his pocket about to see his girl than in the great man with millions about to board his yacht for the South Seas but whose prostate is acting up."

He himself was succeeding, but he was still restless. Only a few months after his arrival in Montreal he told Frances:

> I will stay one year, I think, and then Archibald will be able to place me somewhere.... He has told me he can't hold out any hopes of a hospital appointment here—my appointment is with the university—but I told him I was indifferent to that—all I wanted was a thorough training in chest work—then I can go anywhere.

He had no definite destination. He thought of sanatorium work in England and was considering "a tentative offer from Shanghai." Early in 1929 his interest shifted: "... I must look for a job in the States, I think, in the summer. I shall dislike leaving Montreal, but [I am] feeling my life's rhythm is a determined and pre-destined irregular one, so I accept it." By early spring he was reluctantly preparing to leave Montreal: "This is a lovely town. It's a pity I can't stay but I leave in June—on again—God knows where, not that it matters."

Part of his frustration sprang from his perennial financial problems. He was trying to live on his fellowship and the insurance indemnity, having decided that "I will never return to private practice and am getting prepared to do nothing but chest work." Another problem was his reluctance to accept his position as assistant. As ever, he was eager to lead, not to follow. He had discussed his future with Dr. John Alexander, an eminent thoracic surgeon at the University of Michigan. Alexander had replied,

> As to your own problem for the future, I consider it both a difficult and an easy one, difficult if your health and financial state make it impossible to build up *your own* service in some city during the necessary first lean years; easy because you have had a splendid fundamental training and therefore are well ahead of the men who have not had it and who too often are able by persistence to build up their own services. I agree with what you imply that you are already too far advanced in the field to continue as an assistant.

Unable to strike out on his own, he remained at the Royal Victoria. On March 20, 1930, he received an appointment as Clinical Assistant in Surgery. This was followed five days later by another appointment as a consultant in tuberculosis at Ste. Anne de Bellevue Veterans Hospital. Archibald, in a letter of recommendation, wrote that Bethune had "... been nearly two years with me and I have found him invaluable. A very promising young man." Bethune's financial plight was somewhat eased by a salary of $25.00 which he received for his weekly visit to the government hospital.

The Department of Surgery appointment was explicit recognition by Archibald of Bethune's contributions. There were, however, negative aspects that had begun to irritate both Archibald and others at the Royal Victoria.

Chief among them was Bethune's exasperating tendency to question every concept and opinion of his colleagues and his superiors. Unlike most of them, he openly subjected all clinical and surgical techniques, no matter how fundamental, to rigorous criticism. The more traditional and tried the procedure, the more critical he became. Many staff members felt that Bethune was attacking them personally and not their theories. Certainly when investigation led him to reject the opinions of his colleagues, he made no attempt to conceal his reaction. A friend and physician who later became Physician-in-Chief of the Royal Victoria Hospital stated that Bethune was "critical of things in a healthy . . . but completely outspoken way and he liked to shock people." A colleague pointed out that Bethune " . . . had a good mind, inquiring and honest. But he made enemies because he was so outspoken. [He would] criticize some of his older colleagues with unpardonable rudeness, yet he was quite right because he was really ahead of his time." His direct questioning at staff meetings or medical conventions of Montreal's leading doctors, including his own chief, rankled some of his colleagues:

> He would put forward his own views in an extreme way just to cause discussion . . . . That would arouse antagonism particularly if he were questioning the teaching or the ideas of the senior men, as Archibald was. And quite often the doctors got that idea of him, that he was being too irreverent. Of course everybody loved Archibald. To have him questioned this way wasn't the thing. It never seemed to me that Bethune meant it that way.

His motivation in questioning everything stemmed from a profound and troubling belief that very few persons thought independently. Not only in professional circles but at social gatherings he sparked discussions by taking stands which he really did not support, simply to encourage those around him to think. It appalled him to discover how easily apparently intelligent persons could be swayed by forceful though illogical argument or through sheer intellectual laziness:

He was always the uncommon man in any gathering . . . . I can't say it brought him any particular pride, for, though he enjoyed winning an argument on an unpopular position, he was more often saddened by the uniformity of the complacency that surrounded him, perhaps particularly in his professional life. I like to think of him as a medical cartoonist with . . . bite and punch . . . who could attack any party, any coterie, and any view, but with the same somewhat saddened, wry smile.

At times his mocking manner could turn to cruelty. His friend Louis Huot, at that time a Montreal journalist, said that

He would make a legitimate attempt to make an explanation. Then beyond a certain point he would just engage in the most facetious and mocking sort of comments that only an exceptionally talented person would understand. He would make a fool of his interlocutor, and on purpose.

Unable to conceal his feelings he was hostile in crude and sometimes juvenile ways. He once interrupted a conversation with a friend in a restaurant, explaining that he had just seen someone he particularly disliked and would return as soon as he had "irritated" the offensive party.

He could move from thought to action so quickly and easily that he often confounded others whose minds worked more slowly or more cautiously. No less confounding was his intense concentration. Once he caught the scent of discovery, he seldom rested or ate until he had completed his work. The inability or unwillingness of most of his colleagues to share his extreme enthusiasm earned for them his contempt:

Despite his dedication, impatience and practically manic drive to get things done, he was a surprisingly reasonable and stimulating person to work with. He only became unreasonable and impossible when he thought that someone was not willing to give his best to a cause of investigation that he, Bethune, believed to be important or of benefit to patients or the "underdog."

He was angriest with people who shared his conclusions and lacked his courage to act on them. This was especially true when the powerful force of tradition and custom restrained others, a bond that never held him, and one therefore which he failed to understand. Absorbed by his tubercular research, he became contemptuously resentful of anyone who seemed to frustrate his efforts: "Red tape he detested. Let's get on with the job in hand was more his way of doing things. Direct and to the point type of man...." Added to his innate distrust of authority was a contempt for institutional thinking which appeared to him to place regulations above the essential purpose of the hospital—saving lives. His impatience with individuals and with the rules and regulations of the Royal Victoria Hospital was gradually alienating him from everyone there.

However troubled Bethune's professional life was becoming in 1931, it was nothing compared to the turbulence of his personal life. He refused to accept the loss of Frances as permanent and maintained a correspondence with her in Scotland. In one of his letters to her shortly after his arrival in Montreal, he described his joy at receiving the Cowans Fellowship:

I can scarcely tell you, my darling Frances, how glad [I am] for your sake this fellowship has turned up. That happiness of yours is, to me, the most desired thing in the world. If it were not for my doubts, I would say at once—"Come here. Marry me. Why should we be separate who love each other?" I can be happy with you—but you not with me? I was thinking that if you come here this winter—we could meet just as friends, living apart. In any case whether you marry me or not, that is, I am sure, our only way.... I miss you dreadfully but—I don't want to snatch at you ever again. I want you to be just Frances Penney—without any attempts at approximations to standards, types of my imagination or fancy—the Frances Penney I knew in Edinburgh, self-contained and undistorted.

Your affectionate lover
Beth

He soon became more plaintive:

> It is very pleasant here—very gentle and quiet and I am a different soul. Very clear and cold today. Sun shimmering on the snow and the sparrows making a racket outside my windows. I wish you were here. I am glad you are relatively happy and well, at least more so than when you lived with my petulant irritability.
>
> God bless you
> Beth

Eventually he wore down her resistance and she agreed to return to Canada. At the beginning, their reunion was successful. They decided to remarry in November, 1929, and Bethune appropriately chose Armistice Day for the marriage. In a quiet ceremony in Westmount witnessed by only two friends, the second marriage began. Their happiness was shortlived. They began to quarrel almost immediately and soon discussed divorce. Frances became interested in A.R.E. Coleman, a friend of Bethune, and began to talk with him about the possibility of marriage.

In the autumn of 1931 Bethune went to the southwestern United States on a combined lecture and study tour. From Arizona he wrote Frances:

> I have no desire to force you into marriage with R.E. Believe me, I will never force you to do anything your heart is opposed to, ever again. I love you and always will however much you may hurt or wound me—and now all that is left for me to show you I love you is to help you to gain what you want. I can do that best by keeping you supplied with money, I think . . . . I will not obtain a divorce.

A month later, events had again changed his mind. From Alabama, on New Year's Eve, he wrote to ask for a divorce:

> Well, my dear, the unexpected has happened as usual. I have fallen in love and want to marry this girl that I feel sure I can be happy with. It was love at first sight with both of us . . . .

Darling, let us give up trying to reconcile our irreconcilable natures. As you have said so often, "Breakfast, dinner and bed are not for us two." Our only kinship is a "spiritual affinity" and this, alas, is not enough at our time of life and age . . . . Instead of torturing ourselves with mutual recriminations let us quietly acknowledge the fact and live apart as friends—true friends. We can and will. The affection I feel for you and have felt for you in the past is unique—I can never feel it again for anyone—I am not sure I want to.

You will love her. You are both much the same—the same qualities in you attracted her to me [sic] in the first place—her lovely spirit and mind with the soul of a poet. Will you write her?

. . . since I love and am loved I have lost all the bitterness I felt towards you, darling, and my heart is filled with the warmest affection and regard.

Your friend
Beth

Frances did nothing about this extraordinary letter, and events proved her right. The affair ended as quickly as it began.

In January, 1932, Bethune arrived in Ann Arbor, Michigan, to visit his friend John Barnwell, and to undergo a thorough examination of his lungs. Since his release from Trudeau he had continued to receive regularly a small pneumothorax in his left lung. He used to amaze his friends and even his colleagues by administering the partial collapse himself:

He would come into the ward, ask me for a pneumothorax needle . . . . He never used novocaine on himself. He would open his shirt, stick the needle in his chest, hook up the pneumothorax machine and give himself the air. The machine . . . was his own invention. Then he would go about his business.

Shortly after his arrival at the Royal Victoria Hospital he met Dr. Ronald Christie, who was interested in measuring lung function. He examined Bethune:

I was measuring his lung volume before and after he had a pneumothorax. His pneumothoracies were very small . . . . He had no active tuberculosis . . . . He was having a small pneumothorax on one side that was kept going. He had no temperature. He was perfectly active. He'd take his refill and would be off skiing. As a skier he kept up to any of us.

At Ann Arbor, Dr. John Alexander performed a phrenicectomy on Bethune. In this operation the surgeon opens the neck and cuts the phrenic nerve to paralyze the diaphragm, thereby allowing the lung additional rest. It was usually performed when patients ended their pneumothorax treatments, before the lung re-expanded to assume its normal functions. Bethune's operation became particularly painful when Dr. Alexander, unable to find the accessory fibres, was forced to pull out the nerve. After the operation, with sweat pouring from his forehead, Bethune, who up to this time had made a practice of pulling the nerve, swore he would never do it again.

Coincidentally, Bethune himself had just performed a phrenicectomy. In Arizona he had been asked to treat an aging movie star, Renée Adorée. Before the operation, he devised a necklace to hide the inevitable scar in her neck. He removed several beads from one of Miss Adorée's necklaces, replacing them with a narrow slotted silver bar. When the necklace was fastened around her neck in its natural position, he traced a thin line through the narrow slot. Along this line he made the incision. After the operation, when the beads had been replaced, the necklace concealed the scar. "Strange to say, this seems to fill the female breast with the most profound gratitude," he said later in an article he wrote to collect a wager. After arguing with a colleague that most editors of medical journals were in such awe of so-called experts that they would publish virtually anything written by the big names in thoracic surgery without questioning its literary or scientific merits, he submitted his article describing Miss Adorée's necklace. Bethune won his wager. He later admitted the spoofing nature of the article. Under the heading *Confessional Note,* appended to a 1936 article describing some new surgical instruments, he wrote: "A phrenicectomy necklace described in the Review of Tuberculosis (1932, 23:3) was abandoned as unnecessary. It was taken, as it was meant to be, as an amusing little trinket."

Following his operation, he remained in Ann Arbor with John Barnwell, visiting the hospital and studying the techniques of Dr. Alexander and his staff. He returned to Montreal, where he stayed for only a month before deciding in March to return to Michigan. The Chief of Thoracic Surgery at Detroit's Herman Kieffer Hospital had broken his back in an automobile accident, and Bethune quickly accepted the offer to assume his duties until he recovered. The opportunity to take such an important position, if only temporarily, appealed to him. In addition to gaining valuable surgical experience at Kieffer, he was responsible for tubercular care in sanatoria at Battle Creek and Northville, Michigan.

In the early 1930's, surgical treatment of pulmonary tuberculosis was relatively new in Canada. Lung surgery had been performed as early as the 1890's by German and Swiss surgeons but progress had been slow because of the dangers involved. The purpose of the basic lung operation, the thoracoplasty, was the same as that of the artificial pneumothorax, i.e., to collapse the diseased part of the lung. However, when adhesions joined the lung to the chest wall, pneumothorax was not possible and, in order to permit a collapse of the lung, surgeons removed the ribs of a patient around the diseased area. The operation was usually done in stages depending upon the extent of pulmonary infection. Chief among the problems in this form of surgery was controlling the loss of blood. Another was the necessity to work quickly for fear of keeping the patient under anaesthetic for an unduly long period. A second form of surgical treatment was the lobectomy. Rather than collapse the entire lung, surgeons removed the diseased lobe. In rare cases the removal of an entire lung, a pneumonectomy, was performed.

Bethune learned these types of surgery from Edward Archibald. He soon developed a reputation for speed and dexterity. An intern at the Royal Victoria who assisted Bethune recalls that

> At the beginning of the operation he would mention the time of the clock on the wall. At the completion . . . he again would mention the time. He made an effort to do the operation as rapidly as possible commensurate with safety, and, of course, the purpose of speed was to reduce the time for anaesthesia and period of shock. There was a little criticism of his desire for speed but his motive was the welfare of the patient.

His swiftness astonished some. A surgeon who watched Bethune demonstrate to a group of doctors described his speed:

> The patient . . . was being given a general anaesthetic. After a few minutes the anaesthetist said, "OK, go ahead!" Bethune had already dissected and crushed the nerve. He said, "Stop the anaesthetic, I have just one more skin clip to put in." It was an eye-opener to many of us.

Speed was not the only characteristic of his surgical technique. He was also daring and willing to take risks. "He was not a reformer, he was actually a revolutionary in medical practice," commented a colleague. Some were critical of his surgery, and felt he was a showman, perhaps a poseur. Dr. Arthur Vineberg, a personal friend, recalled an operation at which he assisted:

> He was brilliant, no question about that, and he had technical skills, but the kind of technical skill that kills people because he always liked to go too fast. He did a thoracoplasty for Dr. Archibald in front of a lot of surgeons and he . . . said, "Come on, Arthur, we will show them how good

we are" ... and out came three ribs. I said, "Norman, this
guy is going to bleed to death." "No," he said, "sixteen
minutes from skin to skin!" And the guy died.

Bethune had heard the whispered criticisms in the staff
room but said nothing. When he believed he was wrong,
he confessed his errors. At Detroit's Harper Hospital he
had operated on a woman with a tumour in the lower
abdomen. She told Bethune that the University Clinic in
Hartford, Connecticut, had refused to operate, considering it too dangerous—would he be willing to take the
risk? He accepted. The operation was long and compli-
cated, Bethune ran into trouble, and the patient's leg had
to be amputated. He was distraught, but the Chief Surgeon,
Dr. Berlin, tried to console him by explaining that the operation had been recently performed by an eminent Boston
surgeon with the same result. Bethune then requested permission to explain the operation at a staff meeting. Following Bethune's description, Dr. Berlin rose and told the
meeting what he had told Bethune. A colleague said that
Bethune " ... was in no way held responsible or in poor
regard because of this by the hospital authorities. It was
the measure of the man that he had the courage to
stand up there and say what he did."

At the Royal Victoria, Bethune was convinced that he
was right. He did not have to defend himself. But others,
including Archibald, did not agree, and eventually Archibald questioned Bethune's surgical techniques and his
judgement. Originally the relationship between the two
men had been warm. Archibald referred to Bethune as
"one of the youngest and most brilliant" surgeons in his
service. There were, however, personality differences between the two men which were accentuated in time. Archibald was eighteen years older than Bethune, soft spoken,
slow and careful in his movements. These differences also
appeared in their operating techniques. Archibald was
methodical, cautious and patient. Students used to quip
that once Archibald had made the opening incision, it was
time for the assistants to take tea.

Eventually these contrasting styles led to serious differences of opinion. Bethune believed that most postoperative deaths were attributable to surgical shock from keeping the patient under anaesthetic too long. He once remarked impatiently to an intern after they had watched Archibald take more than two hours to perform a lobectomy that the operation could be done in only three-quarters of an hour. The intern recalls, "My quiet reaction was that this was so much malarkey until, about a week later, Bethune booked a lobectomy and with only my assistance completed the performance in just under an hour." His decision to increase his operating speed may, in some cases, have led to less attention in his handling of tissues and other structures. A clinical clerk described the situation:

> I became aware that Dr. Bethune's patients had a rocky time recovering from surgery, more frequently than those of Dr. Archibald or Dr. McIntosh. It was not a problem of infection . . . but poor general physical condition on their return from the operating room and shock . . . . In spite of our best care we were losing patients operated on by Dr. Bethune at an unusual rate.

Archibald spoke to Bethune but they could not agree and Bethune persisted in his surgical approach. When one of Bethune's patients who had been considered a good risk failed to survive a first-stage thoracoplasty, Archibald and Bethune clashed. Shortly after the encounter, Bethune left the Royal Victoria Hospital.

Archibald later said of Bethune that "he was a leader, but . . . a dangerous kind of leader—certainly dangerous in regard to t.b. and surgery. He was willing to take risks at the patient's expense . . . ." Much more than professional differences separated the two men. Archibald stated: "I never really liked him; our outlook on life was too dissimilar." He found Bethune " . . . definitely abnormal, but not 'mental' and not a genius nor a leader . . . . He was an egocentric, his vision was keen but narrow. He wore blinkers. He trod on many toes quite often without knowing it or without caring if he did know it. He had a superiority complex and he was entirely amoral." Bethune once startled Archibald at a social event by stating, "Oh, what's the use. I will never manage to explain anything to you. The trouble is that, by nature, you shoot butterflies with a shotgun and I like to hunt elephants with a bow and arrow."

Others have disagreed with Archibald's evaluation of Bethune's surgery:

> Norman was what I would consider an excellent operator and . . . exhibited sound surgical judgement. . . . His philosophy was that every open case of t.b. was responsible for at least ten more. He therefore felt that high risk procedures were justified in the endeavour to convert every open case of t.b. . . .
> He was a very impulsive individual in both his professional and social activities. His opinions were quickly made *probably* without complete knowledge of the particular situation but peculiarly enough it [sic] was usually right. This impulsive attitude frequently annoyed Dr. Archibald and his confrères.

There is little doubt that his impulsive nature and his stubborn self-reliance at times affected his judgement, but the charge that because of a commitment to pure science and an eagerness for self-glorification he treated his patients as guinea pigs has no foundation. A McGill medical student who assisted him with a thoracoplasty remembers that "he worked with skill and despatch and his attitude made me aware that it was a patient he was operating on, not a case of tuberculosis." A nurse described Bethune's attitude towards his patients:

> He was very keenly interested in those patients with tuberculosis. His sympathy and concern for them was always very evident. They were individuals and not something or someone whom he could experiment on. A patient he operated on became almost his personal possession. He

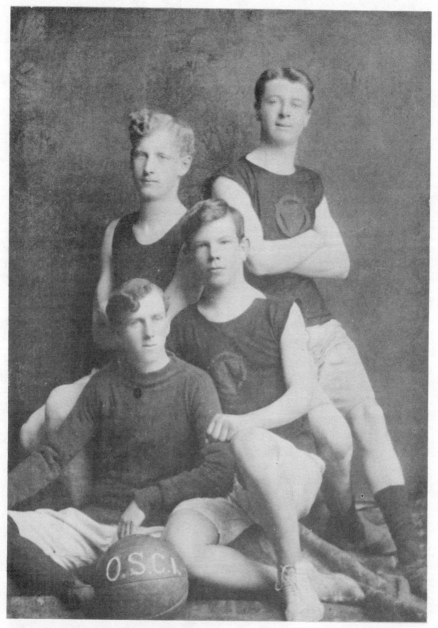

Norman Bethune (second from the right) age 14 or 15, with three other members of the Owen Sound Collegiate Institute soccer team. They are (clockwise from right rear) Lewis, McNeil and Clark.

He was born in 1890 in the clap-
board Presbyterian manse on John
Street in Gravenhurst, Ontario.
The photograph was taken in
1972.

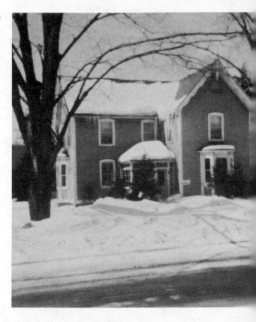

Bethune (centre) worked north of
Georgian Bay for Frontier College
in 1910–11.

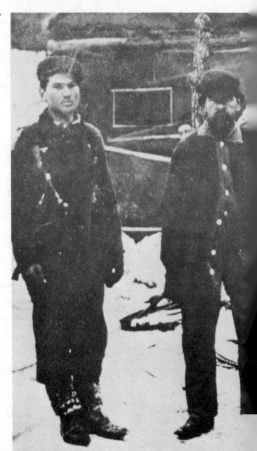

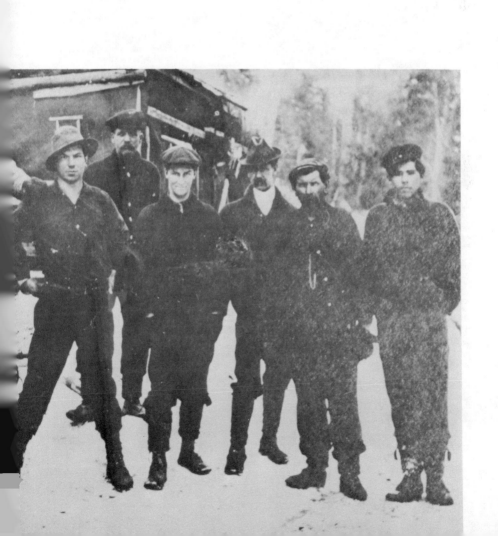

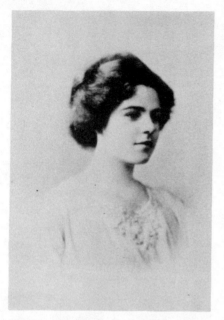 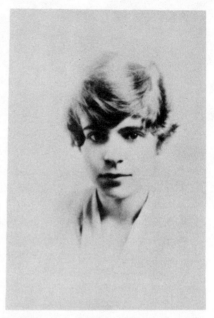

Frances Campbell Penney, later Bethune's wife, in her teens.

Frances, probably around the age of 20.

Bethune was at Trudeau Sanatorium in 1927 with (left to right) Dr. Lincoln Fisher, Dr. John Barnwell, Dr. Alfred Blalock, and an unknown friend.

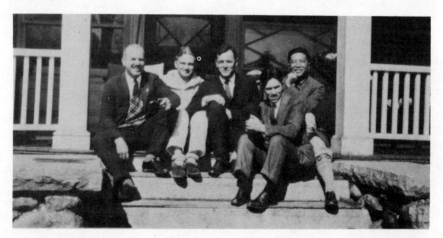

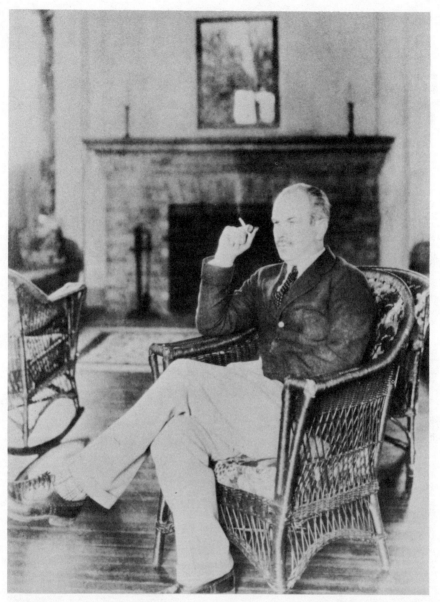

Sanatorium regulations forbade smoking, but Bethune paid no attention.

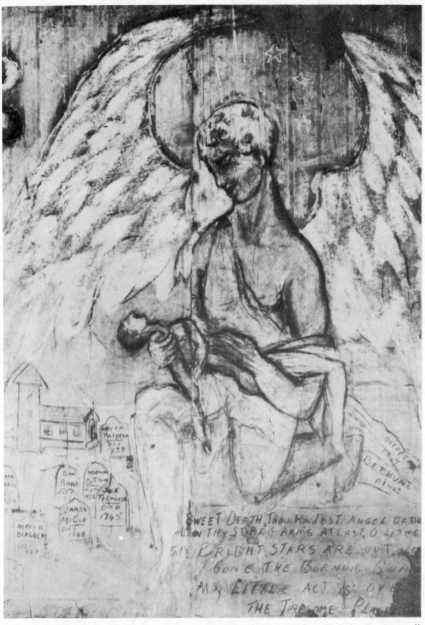

In the final panel of his mural at Trudeau, "The T.B.'s Progress", Bethune painted himself in the arms of the Angel of Death. He tried to predict his own death date on the tombstone at lower left, but actually lived until 1939.

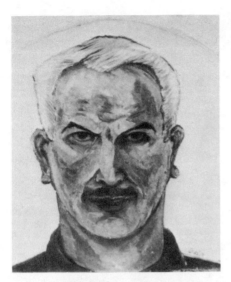

His self-portrait in oils, painted in 1935, was later presented by McGill University to the people of China on McGill's Bethune Day, November 25, 1971.

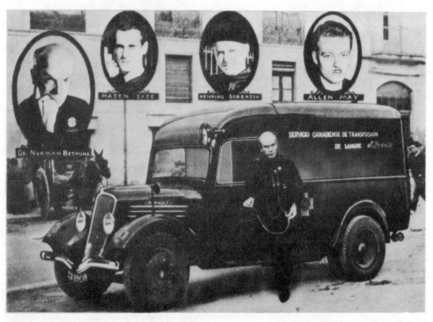

Bethune drove the Renault truck on the rescue mission to Malaga in February, 1937. From the left, his companions in Madrid were Hazen Sise and Henning Sorensen, both of Montreal, and Allen May of Toronto.

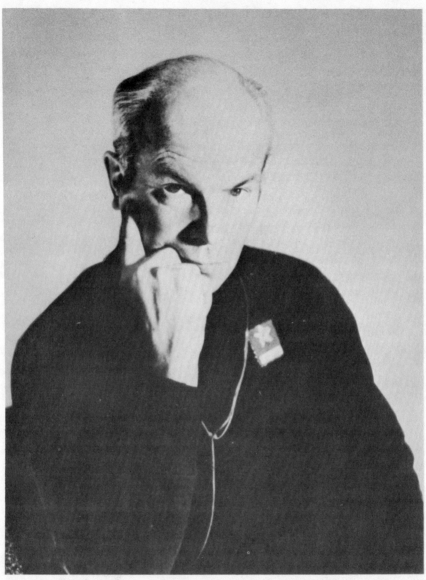

Bethune, a good photographer himself, liked to be photographed. He sent copies of this picture from Madrid to his friends in Canada in early 1937.

would visit a patient 2-3 times a day until they were well
on the way to recovery, delighted when they did well, always
serious and always encouraging them. When complications
would arise, he would become very upset and never stop
worrying . . .

One of his assistants was convinced Bethune always put
his patients first:

> After an operation he used to go and see the patients more
> often than he was supposed to do, because he was extremely
> devoted to his patients. Of course, like any surgeon, he
> lost patients, but I couldn't stay around when he lost a
> patient because he was so sorry. He was very unhappy when
> he lost a patient . . . .He would cry or be mad.

Henning Sorensen, his interpreter in Spain, most accur-
ately described his relationship with his patients: "He was
like a father. There was actually, in this man with a big
ego, there was love, and they felt it. He communicated
it to the wounded. And he was very concerned. He was
so excited when they recovered."

Bethune was daring, impulsive and impatient. As one
of his former students remarked, " . . . he was a hell of
a good surgeon, there is no doubt about that. Fast and
brilliant and occasionally he made mistakes. Of course,
we remember the mistakes." Yet the mistakes resulted from
his attempt to save lives. Any significant medical advance
results from imaginative and daring acts and, because most
doctors are not willing to take risks, they tend to be critical
and even hostile to the daring. Another of his students
said, "Anyone who is ahead of the crowd in medicine is
noted as using his patients as guinea pigs."

The final rupture with Archibald did not surprise
Bethune. He had long been aware of his professional and
personal image at the Royal Victoria. To some he was
a dangerous rebel whose reckless surgical style and unconventional social manner were incongruous with the highly
conservative atmosphere of Montreal's leading hospital.
To others he was a highly skilled surgeon whose concern

for his patients, combined with his perceptive discovery of and willingness to practise new ideas, more than balanced his eccentric personal ways. Among those who felt uneasy in his presence and who rejected his style of life, his departure was a blessing. Their attitude was succinctly expressed by a colleague: "He didn't fit in here."

The variety of opinions is understandable. Bethune was a man of contradictions. His swiftly changing moods frequently led to alternating courses of action which baffled all but the very few who knew him. Dr. Aubrey Geddes, a physician at the Royal Victoria who shared an apartment with Bethune for more than a year, described his dress: "He was a conservative person, a stickler for form, always very correctly dressed, his clothes bought from the most expensive tailor in town....[He was] always insisting on white tie and tails at every appropriate occasion." At other times he would be the opposite, seemingly unconcerned about the clothes he was wearing. His style of dress was well in advance of his time. When most medical doctors were wearing suits, Bethune often dressed in grey slacks, sport jacket and coloured shirt, or a beret and turtleneck sweater. Once he went out to a party with a friend wearing shoes, trousers and overcoat but no shirt or jacket. On another occasion, apparently on a dare, he did his ward rounds dressed as a lumberjack.

He responded to dares. During a New Year's Eve party in the Laurentians, he was talking about the effect of cold on the human body. When someone suggested that no one could remain in the river outside the cottage for as long as a minute, he scoffed. Someone else offered to bet he was wrong. He stood up, accepted the wager, walked out the door and into the river where he remained for the required minute. Back in the cabin and obviously numbed, he sat steaming before the fire without speaking. He had proved his point.

Bethune was readily distinguishable from his colleagues. Wearing a green pork-pie hat and a scarf around his neck, he drove his yellow roadster at high speed through the streets of Montreal. His sense of humour was clever and sometimes bizarre. In order to cure a patient who insisted

his stomach pains were caused by a frog he had swallowed,
Bethune came to the hospital with a frog in his pocket,
gave the patient an enema, then slipped the frog into the
pan and showed it to him. The stomach pains vanished.
Bethune speculated that in his mental condition the man
would likely return with a more challenging ailment, but
he had at least given him temporary relief. In the bathroom
of his apartment he kept four cans of different coloured
paint. Friends were invited to dip a hand into the paint
and press it to the wall, leaving an imprint. Then, with
a paint-covered forefinger, the friend wrote his or her name
in the space left by the palm. The yellow bathroom
wall was covered with a maze of bright autographed hands.
  His social attitudes were equally paradoxical. He was

  ... an aristocrat by nature. He was proud of what he called
  his aristocratic lineage, fond of talking about the Bethunes
  of France who date back to William the Conqueror and
  before. And he often quoted the line of the Four
  Marys—"Mary Queen of Scots, Mary Bethune, Mary Sed-
  don, Mary Carmichael and me." And he always claimed
  lineage from Mary Bethune.

Nevertheless, he openly mocked class distinctions and was
usually much happier in the company of his students or
among artists than in the social circles of most of his colleagues.
  His universal curiosity and intense commitment involved
him in a variety of interests. He had a showy confidence
in his own abilities:

  Norm had a theory that he (or anyone) could do anything
  he wanted to. He said he could paint a picture and have
  it accepted in the Spring Exhibition at the Art Museum.
  So he doggedly painted—and his picture, Night Operating
  Room, was hung in the art show. Having proved that he
  went on to something else.

Sometimes his self-assurance extended him beyond his
limits. He decided to write a definitive monograph on the
physical signs of tuberculosis, an area in which he had

little training. After he had completed it, he asked for a colleague's criticisms:

> ... I sat down and it took me about half an hour to read it. I scribbled in the margin all the way down, "not proved," "unknown," "hypothesis" and so on. I went over it with him and he said, "Ronald, you are absolutely right." ... He got up in his theatrical way and he tore this manuscript in small bits, chucked it in the wastepaper basket and said, "Now let's go and have a drink." That is the last I heard of it and he had spent weeks on it.

He rarely treated failure this lightly—more often it led to frustration and anger. After working intensely for several days on a painting of a world of breasts with a small man lying among them, he gave up and destroyed the painting.

Above all he wanted to live life significantly and vividly. Unlike most men who sense the mystery of life but are awed by it, Bethune actively set out to unlock the secret doors, Marian Scott, a close friend from Montreal, termed him

> ... one of the most alive and aware people. [He was] very anxious to live his life well .... He would talk about the destructive things in his life, but he also felt that deep conviction...[of] a perception or intuition of some kind of truth. He called it a vision ....He had a great belief... about something to follow in life ... some kind of evolving reality. He believed we were part of a kind of adventure of living, that we couldn't tell after we had gone what was coming, but each one of us perhaps could do something towards a direction of the one sense—he called it intuition.

In his search for the one sense, he was forever breaking the chains of convention and tradition that seemed to him to imprison not only most men's actions but also their thoughts:

> He had a great impatience with what most people would feel was everyday life. One of the things he found hardest

to bear was ordinariness or mundaneness. He was always longing to live every hour intensely and . . . he felt that life was going on at too slow a pace. This was quite apart from his feeling of compassion and wanting to do something about it. Often he would . . . seem to people to be almost anxious to shock which would be partly a suffocated feeling he had that our society was so routine, so regimented, and that we didn't really even realize what we were ourselves.

There was more than a routine pattern to people's lives. There was waste and emptiness. He felt this especially of the wealthy who were cocooned in their tiny world, ignorant of or indifferent toward others. To Bethune there was a circular repetitiveness to the life style of many of the members of his own profession and the businessmen and lawyers with whom they associated. Despite their education, they were insensitive, dull and unaware. This irritation often triggered his caustic and Rabelaisian wit.

As a dinner party guest in a wealthy Montreal home he ridiculed the fetish of body cleanliness and suggested that the animal odours of human bodies were stimulating and pleasant. One woman, totally unaware that Bethune was performing, turned to him in astonishment and asked, "But . . . if we didn't bathe, how could we remain clean?" Bethune paused, leaned across the table, and said in a bored manner, "Oh . . . I don't know . . . we might just lick each other clean."

On another occasion, again a dinner party, Bethune appeared in dinner jacket, accompanied by a prostitute. He paraded her before the awe-struck guests, took her to the buffet table, filled her plate with food and handed her a drink. When she had finished, he announced to the silent onlookers, "Now, ladies and gentlemen, I shall return her whence she has come—the streets and degradation."

This type of behaviour achieved the intended effect of shocking, and it also made Bethune increasingly unpopular in polite society. Moreover, the premeditated manner often explicit in his behaviour seemed to mitigate the satisfaction he derived from these outbursts. His compulsive actions were usually followed by regret: "If I could only repress my irritating delight in shocking the timid, I think I might learn to be decent too," he once confessed to Frances. In his desire to be natural, to be himself, he tried to maintain an inner integrity while ignoring the rules of standard social behaviour. The two were in direct conflict.

To his friends he was warm and generous. An artist described him as "... a rock. [He had] that essence that D.H. Lawrence speaks of, that kind of inner quality in a man which you have to search down for and find .... Perhaps a lot of people have that essence and quality but it doesn't show very much. With Bethune it showed." This quality revealed itself in his passionate and open desire to help others. When a friend complimented him on his wool overcoat, Bethune took it off and offered it as a gift. The friend remarked: "I did not accept it ... but he was very generous.... He hadn't any sense of ownership.... Anything that he owned, he would give to his friends. He bought some paintings by different artists and he gave them away ... to his friends." He asked an artist friend, Fritz Brandtner, to design a book plate which read "This book belongs to Norman Bethune and his friends." A fast reader, he bought hundreds of books, glued the book plate in each, read them and gave them away.

He always loved to give and to receive presents. When he returned from Europe, he came back loaded with gifts for members of his family. His gifts were not always expensive. Usually acting on inspiration, he would buy simple presents, a wooden spoon that caught his eye in Woolworth's or a children's book that appealed to him. However, the erratic nature of his giving would sometimes anger and confuse friends. He once gave a book to a friend and took it back a few days later, explaining that it had only been "a gift for lend."

He was spontaneous, warming quickly to a subject, concentrating all of his energies on it for a sustained period of time and then losing interest as quickly as he had gained it. During his campaign against tuberculosis he persuaded

Fritz Brandtner to design a model city for tuberculars. He and Brandtner spent days together planning. When Bethune returned from a trip he never again mentioned the subject to Brandtner. It had vanished from his mind to be replaced by some other scheme.

The contradictions were tolerated by some and understood by few, least of all by his colleagues. He began to feel ostracized and gradually found acquaintances among artists and writers. In 1931 he attended art classes held by Adam Sheriff Scott, who remembers that Bethune attended only irregularly and worked on his own. Scott felt that Bethune had a natural ability which allowed him to develop in a very brief period of time. But, as usual, Bethune was drawn away by other interests. From October, 1931, to August, 1932, he was in Montreal for fewer than two months. He never attended formal art classes again but his growing camaraderie with artists sustained his interest and during his remaining years in Montreal he continued to paint periodically.

By the beginning of 1933 he had reached another plateau. He had lost his position at the Royal Victoria, his second marriage was a continuing disaster, and, as usual, he was broke.

I am an Artist

Bethune returned from Ann Arbor in February, 1932, and began to look for another position. The future break with Archibald could be predicted by all concerned, and Bethune himself was restless—he had been at the Royal Victoria for five years, the longest unbroken service in his career. He learned that Sacré Coeur Hospital was looking for a qualified surgeon to direct their new tubercular unit. Archibald, despite their differences, suggested Bethune for the position, and, in September, his name was placed in nomination before the Medical Bureau of the hospital.

When Archibald dismissed Bethune in the fall of 1932, his search for work became more urgent. In the eyes of the Montreal medical establishment, a rupture with Archibald was unpardonable. As one Montreal doctor said, "The Royal Victoria was the ivory tower and once you start going to the Women's General and places like that, you are on the down slide."* On November 26, following an interview with Bethune, the Sister Superior announced to the Medical Bureau that he had accepted the position.

*Bethune received a part-time appointment at Women's General Hospital in 1934.

Following his first operation at Sacré Coeur on January 30, 1933, Bethune wrote:

> Ten miles from Montreal—French Canadian and Catholic, twelve hundred dollars a year, one day a week, so the strain is less strained. I cauterized some adhesions there yesterday, and the chorus of oh's and ah's from the nuns rose like a chant at the high altar. My title is "Chef dans le Service de Chirurgie Pulmonaire et de Bronchoscopie." I'm going to have a nice big white cap made with "Chef" marked in front. Really, I'm delighted.

The appointment was extremely important to Bethune. At last he had realized one of his most desired goals—he was in charge of his own service. One of the conditions of the appointment was that Bethune would train an assistant. During his stay of almost four years he took on two: Dr. Georges Deshaies, who eventually succeeded him, and Dr. Gérard Rolland. Bethune did much for Sacré Coeur. Since he was an internationally known doctor, colleagues came to view his work, and he helped develop the reputation of the institution.

This was a productive time for Bethune as surgeon and teacher. His odd behaviour, his perpetual demand for perfection, and his impatience all remained, but his relationship with the hospital officials, the nursing sisters and the medical doctors was more warm and cordial than it had been at the Royal Victoria. Now that he had his own service he could make his own decisions. He felt that he was being recognized, that he was considered useful. Dr. Georges Cousineau, the anaesthetist for most of his operations, said: "He was for all of us an inspiration in his work and his research and during these ... years among us he never stopped teaching and inspiring each and every one of us to do more and more careful work."

Bethune's eccentricities sometimes confused and sometimes awed his colleagues at Sacré Coeur. After a fire in his apartment had destroyed most of his possessions including all his clothes, Bethune appeared at the hospital wearing an old suit and shoes with no soles—as usual, he didn't have enough money to buy a new suit. Dr. Cousineau knew that Bethune refused to send bills to his few private patients. Bethune said himself that if he were to establish a private practice, he would place a box near the door and as a patient left he could show his appreciation by putting a little money in the box. Cousineau was concerned by Bethune's situation and approached the director of the hospital to obtain a list of Bethune's patients:

> Then I made a collection among his patients and . . . collected $300. The following day he returned better dressed but without a cent. [He said] "Georges, lend me five bucks." He had in fact bought himself some clothes but he had also divided the money among those poor children to whom he taught painting.

His international reputation grew during his period at Sacré Coeur Hospital. In 1932 he had been elected an associate member of the American Association of Thoracic Surgery. He was often invited to the National Tuberculosis and Canadian Medical Association Conferences to read his papers and offer his opinions because he was interesting and controversial: " . . . he presented certain scientific papers at the programs in a most unusual fashion, one which had a great impact on his audience. He was unusual in that he allowed a great deal more of personal expression in his presentations than most of us would permit ourselves." He attacked the giants of international surgery just as he had once criticized experienced Montreal specialists on medical theory. At an afternoon session of the A.A.T.S.,

> there was a series of papers by the biggest names in thoracic surgery showing very low mortality from thoracoplasty operations. Most discussions praised the surgeons, but Bethune criticized them thoroughly. He said they had selected favourable cases to make good statistics [and] had refused operations to many patients whose lives might have been saved. This produced a reaction in [the] Society and many of them became permanent enemies of Bethune because he was taking this attitude toward their work.

In 1935, Bethune became a full member of the A.A.T.S. and was elected to the five-man Council of the society, an impressive tribute to a young man who had entered the field less than seven years earlier.

Each medical conference provided him with an opportunity to preach the gospel of collapse (compression) therapy. His "Compressionist's Creed," as he called it, amused some doctors and irritated others:

I believe in Trudeau the mighty father of the American Sanatorium, maker of a heaven on earth for the tuberculous; and in Artificial Pneumothorax, which was conceived by Carson, born of the labors of Forlanini, suffered under Pompous Pride and Prejudice, was criticized by the Cranks whose patients are dead and buried; thousands now well, even in the third stage, rose again from their bed; ascending into the Heaven of Medicine's Immortals, they sit on the right hand of Hippocrates our Father; from thence they do judge those pthisiotherapists quick to collapse cavities or dead on their job.

I believe in Bodington, Brehmer, Koch and Brauer, in Murphy, Friedrich, Wilms, Sauerbruch, Stuertz and Jacobeus, in the unforgiveness of the sins of omission in Collapse Therapy, in the resurrection of a healthy body from a diseased one and long life for the tuberculous with care everlasting. Amen.

Bethune had sketched the original outline of the prayer during his plane trip from Arizona to Michigan in January, 1932. When he arrived at John Barnwell's home, an Episcopal rectory Barnwell had rented, he conceived the idea of paralleling the Apostle's Creed. He sat in the rector's study with the prayer book open and penned his Compressionist's Creed. Bethune had no desire to be blasphemous. Barnwell pointed out that "it was a time of great despondency both by patients and by doctors, when bed rest was the chief reliance .... He thought it best to offer us all faith and hope by putting his ideas into the form of a profession or a creed of faith."

The sincerity of his commitment, the originality of his approach and the zeal with which he conducted his campaign for collapse therapy attracted the attention of leading international chest surgeons. Many considered him theatrical, rebellious and dangerously iconoclastic, while others saw him as a dramatic and fascinating character, "an enthusiast.... [He was like] an Elizabethan, possibly a rather swashbuckling Elizabethan, and he certainly should have been very successful in the era of Queen Elizabeth." Still others saw, perhaps only dimly, the inner conflict in Bethune. One surgeon described him as "a restless soul wandering in and out of meetings looking for something which I suppose he never found."

His success at Sacré Coeur and his growing international reputation were scarce compensation for the disaster of his second marriage to Frances. Although his affair in Alabama had ended, he was still resolved to divorce her: "I am sorry I came back and disturbed Frances' peace of mind, however. She is beginning to waver but I can see no other way out except to go through with it. I feel that I will eventually destroy not only myself but anyone intimately connected with me." In the summer of 1932 he and Frances decided to seek a divorce. According to Canadian law, adultery had to be established as the cause. Bethune, Frances and A.R.E. Coleman, whom she married several months later, carefully planned the evidence and when the divorce was granted on March 30, 1933, the three celebrated together with champagne.

For both, the divorce was the result of their frustration at living together, but Bethune was still unhappy. He never ceased believing that some relationship could be maintained: to Coleman, whom he had apparently accepted as Frances' future husband, he said, "I don't give away my wife, I only lend her." His feelings about the divorce were very ambivalent. Bethune had asked Louis Huot, a close friend, to appear as a witness, but instead of thanking him, Bethune's first words were, "You are coming between me and the woman I really love in a positive and definitive way." Less than two weeks after the divorce had been granted, Bethune wrote Frances:

I enclose a letter of Millar, Horne & Hanna, the official hangmen. Well, they may think they have done the job but how surprised [they] would be to know that all their mumblings and posturings have left the 2 principals—like 2 naughty, reprimanded boys—sniggling behind their backs.

> God bless you. I love you. Beth

Even after Frances remarried, they saw one another and wrote often.* Although he felt strongly about several women, and proposed to at least two of them, his attachment to Frances remained firm until his death. The failure with her was the greatest in Bethune's life. Despite his very real and profound feeling for her, his desire to dominate, bend and shape her doomed the marriage. He admitted this in a letter written to Frances almost a year after the divorce:

Truthfully and sincerely I believe I want nothing more from you. Not I as a man physically, nor as a soul spiritually. I believe we have had all the profitable commerce between us that is possible, and nothing more is to be gained by prolongation of our relationship. It never at any time completely satisfied either of us—let us make no more attempts. I regret nothing of the past that has happened between us except one thing—my essential masculine stupidity on the non-recognition of reality—and my fumbling attempts to change a fantasy into a fact.

Forgive me, if you can. I am truly sorry for the unhappiness I have caused you. I was like a clumsy and furious gardener, hacking away at a tree, a living tree, in an attempt to make it conform to a preconceived and fantastic design

*Bethune and Frances shared a doll, symbolic, perhaps, of their childless marriage. Frances said later, "Did you know we had a doll-child called Alice? She spent six months with her father and six months with her mother like all good children of divorcees. Beth burnt her up once when he set his room on fire here in Montreal." Of her relationship with Bethune she said, "I left Beth oftener than he left me . . . . [The] first time I divorced but next time we decided fair play meant him doing it. We meant to have a third time. A third marriage or stay put . . ."

of his own. I tried to bend you, to re-make you, not recognizing you as you are, but only with the sort of genetic, stupid male idea of you as woman, any woman—and not as *a* woman, a special kind of woman called Frances Campbell Penney. I know now you must be taken only as you are. You are not to be changed. Either a man must take you as you are or he will destroy both you and himself in the attempt to change you . . . .

I am not going to do that. I believe you must be left alone and then you will flower in peace and quiet and give peace and quietness to those about you. But no persuasion, no aggression of others, and on your part, most important, no attempt to change yourself to please another.

There would be no need for us to part completely if R.E. would abandon his suspicions—suspicions of both you and I. I am not the cause of the disharmony between you two. I am no rival. He has nothing to fear from me. He has only to fear himself. He said at your marriage he accepted the idea of the spiritual relationship between you and I. He must accept it, or it will destroy him. He must accept what you and I have been to each other in the past. It does him no harm. Only egotism forbids acceptance of this.

And you must spend your life acting in the true, internal deep compulsion of your own spirit. You must give up trying to conform to another's idea of you. Do as I do—if I can say that—be yourself and *don't try to please people.* For you that only results in self-mutilation. If they do not accept you as you are—remove yourself, let them go—or go yourself. Only live with those who respect the spiritual and physical necessities of your nature.

The tragedy of it all is this—that between the two of us—R.E. and . myself—two men who protest they love you—we have torn you, violated you and will, if we persist in our present course, distort or destroy one of the sweetest natures that God ever made. Well, I will do my part—I will leave you alone.

I accept gratefully what you once gave me, and now ask you nothing more. That is the only way I can show I love you. I can do nothing for you except leave you alone, entirely. We must die to each other. For peace between you and R.E. you and I must die to each other. Let us remember it only as a dream.

Good-bye, my sweet Frances. I loved you once and to prove it, I will leave you now. Let us part. Good-bye.

Beth

P.S. Show this letter to R.E. I have written it as truthfully and sincerely as I am able. A truthful and sincere soul will accept it as such.

B.

Bethune often drank too much in these years, and would become objectionable and even intolerable to his companions. An artist friend recalls:

When I first met Beth I was drawn to him by his keen intelligence, forceful personality and intensity, but quite quickly I came to regard him as a menace and to actually resent him . . . . He was a bad drinker, that is, as he drank he became increasingly irascible and difficult . . . . Beth loved [to play poker] . . . in a somewhat domineering manner . . . . And so it frequently fell to my lot to cope with him when he had been drinking and was exhibiting the least favourable aspects of himself. He picked arguments and insulted people everywhere we went and got into many more or less serious squabbles. Beth knew that I had been the Canadian Intercollegiate Heavyweight Boxing Champion and as I was a good deal bigger than he was, he was careful never to pick on me. But it devolved upon me to get him out of a good many fights, some of them quite nasty, and to get him home.

After the divorce he shared an apartment with his colleague, Dr. Aubrey Geddes. Both loved parties and the apartment was frequently filled with doctors, artists, writers and poets who would stay half the night, drinking and talking about a great variety of subjects. Bethune usually made himself the centre of attraction at these gatherings:

. . . he delighted in the clash of minds and would go to almost any length to pull a brilliant *bon mot* . . . . We had a large sitting room, and one wall of it . . . was used to write down the *bons mots* that occurred during conversation and the wall was covered after the first year.

He was reading D.H. Lawrence and beginning to write poetry and short stories, but during most of his spare time he painted in an attempt to sort out his many contradictory ideas. "Painting and writing were very important to him. He would often say, 'I am an artist,' meaning that he felt the same way when he was operating as he would feel in working with a canvas. These things were for him closely related." His personal interpretation of the meaning of art reveals that he saw himself more as a feeling than an intellectual person—intuition was Bethune's favourite word for the creative faculty. Art was

> . . . very mysterious, very strange, [the] natural product of the subconscious mind of man, of all men, in some degree. Arising into the realm of deliberate thought, its life is imperilled . . . . A theory of art is an attempt of the rational mind to impose its discipline and its order on the seeming chaos and seeming disorder of the emotional subconscious. If this is attempted . . . a certain form of art, ordered and neat, arises. By its subjection to the conscious mind . . . it lives for a while and then languishes and dies. It can not survive its separation from its great breeding ground of the subconscious. The mind (that alien in the attic) by its dictatorship destroys the very thing it has discovered.
>
> Most great artists of the world have been—thank Heaven—"stupid" in the worldly sense. They didn't think too much, they simply painted. Driven on by an irresistible internal compulsion, they painted as they did, as they must paint.

In his description of the role of the artist he describes, in part, his own view of himself, and revels in the didactics of the amateur:

> A great artist lets himself go. He is natural. He swims easily in the stream of his own temperament. He listens to himself.

He respects himself. He has a deeper fund of strength to draw from than that arising from rational and logical knowledge.

He comes up into the light of every day, like a great leviathan of the deep, breaking the smooth surface of accepted things, gay, serious, sportive and destructive. In the bright, banal glare of day, he enjoys the purification of violence, the catharsis of action. His appetite for life is enormous. He enters eagerly into the life of man, of all men. He becomes all men in himself. He views the world with an all-embracing eye which looks upwards, outwards, inwards and downwards, understanding, critical, tender and severe. Then he plunges back once more, back into the depths of that other world, strange, mysterious, secret and alone. And there, in those depths, he gives birth to the children of his being—new forms, new colours, new wounds, new movements reminiscent of the known, yet not the known; alike and yet unalike; strange yet familiar; calm, profound and sure.

The function of the artist is to disturb. His duty is to arouse the sleeper, to shake the complacent pillars of the world. He reminds the world of its dark ancestry, shows the world its present, and points the way to its new birth. He is at once the product and the preceptor of his time. After his passage we are troubled and made unsure of our too-easily accepted realities. He makes uneasy the static, the set and the still. In a world terrified of change, he preaches revolution—the principle of life. He is an agitator, a disturber of the peace—quick, impatient, positive, restless and disquieting. He is the creative spirit of life working in the soul of men.

Bethune's own painting suffered from his desire "to shake the complacent pillars of the world." His compulsive urge to broaden his interests, and his inability, therefore, to restrict himself to a narrow field prevented him from obtaining what he described as basic needs of the artist, "leisure, immense quietness, privacy and aloneness." The results of the few moments he could spare for painting revealed qualities far beyond the average painter. His works were powerful and intense, dominated by darkness.

Had he given himself the time and possessed the necessary self-discipline, he could have become an excellent artist.

Instead of thoroughly pursuing his own interest in art he tried to develop skills in others. Early in 1936 he rented a third-floor apartment in downtown Montreal overlooking the lower town and the St. Lawrence River. Lonely there sometimes and missing affection, he suggested to Fritz Brandtner that his apartment become a studio in which Brandtner and others would give lessons, at Bethune's expense, to children who could not afford to pay. In the late summer of 1936, the Montreal Children's Creative Art Centre began with classes three afternoons a week and Saturday mornings. Marian Scott, who was one of the instructors, described Bethune's rationale:

> Beth always had this very strong feeling that the children... who were having such a difficult life at the time of the Depression, that if even for a short time each week they could come and work with colours and be free to draw and express their ideas or feelings, that this might even affect them later on when they faced hardships.

Under Fritz Brandtner's direction the children were urged to release their creative energy. First they were taken on expeditions to various parts of the city where they sketched factories, buildings and people in parks and on city streets. On their return they were provided with paints and large sheets of paper which they spread on the floor. A student who later became a professional painter remembered her reaction to the classes: "For the first time in my life I heard someone say, 'Just go ahead and paint what you want to, whatever you like doing best.' In those days the schools didn't have that system. I would say that this was the tone of the school.... You did just what you liked best and the results were really good." The school attracted considerable attention in Montreal and the expressive works of the young children were exhibited at several public showings.

Although he had sometimes expressed radical political

ideas for the sake of argument, Bethune's politics were
anti-establishment in a quite conservative way. Until the
early 1930's he had shown little interest in politics and
government. His friend George Mooney, who met him
in 1933, considered him "a left-wing Tory . . . [who] gradually progressed to a sort of centre position and
then . . . moved toward a general left position." As late as
1934 his ideas were right of centre. According to George
Holt, who once engaged him in a heated argument on
a labour-management question and tried in vain to dis-
suade him from his anti-labour standpoint, there was, in
Bethune's thinking, "a tendency, very definitely, to be a
right-winger." During that same year he met the artists
Jean and Jori Palardy, whom he later described to Marian
Scott as being "too political for me." Jean Palardy remembers that Bethune in 1934 was "anti-socialist."

The first stirrings of his political conscience were closely
associated with his understanding of the social role of medicine. His clinical research discoveries and his surgery led
him to imagine a glorious and beautiful paradise where
disease had been eliminated. In his impatient effort to
create that paradise he viewed every obstacle as a reaction-
ary and malign force. When he began to believe that
through massive and concerted action tuberculosis could
be eliminated he preached this idea to friends and colleagues. He believed that tuberculosis could be almost entirely eradicated by preventive techniques. This to him
would be far superior as an artistic achievement than the
patchwork of surgery. But as his own personal efforts in
this direction did not seem sufficient, he focused more
attention on society rather than on the individual. In 1932,
he described the "close embrace of economics and patho-
logy" in an article:

> The treatment of pulmonary tuberculosis involves two
> problems. The first is that of the infected individual, re-
> garded as a whole, acting and reacting in his social and
> physical environment, and the second, the reaction of that
> individual's body, and more particularly his lungs, to the
> presence of the tubercle bacillus. The tubercle bacillus may

be considered, as it truly is, just another factor in the environment of man, impinging on him, causing certain changes in his body and modifying its behaviour. The first problem then becomes chiefly an economic and social one, and second, a physiological one. In the final analysis, they are mutually reactive and inseparable. Trudeau well said, "there is a rich man's tuberculosis and a poor man's tuberculosis." The rich man recovers and the poor man dies . . . . Lack of time and money kills more cases of pulmonary tuberculosis than lack of resistance to that disease. The poor man dies because he cannot afford to live. Here the economist and the sociologist meet the compressionist on common ground.

Not content with the effort to interest his own profession in his ideas, Bethune began to make public speeches. In 1934, speaking to the Canadian Progress Club of Montreal, he conducted an imaginary investigation of the circumstances surrounding the death of John Bunyan, a victim of tuberculosis. After an examination by a doctor who used only a stethoscope, Bunyan became progressively more ill. A second doctor, with the aid of an x-ray machine, discovered that Bunyan had pulmonary tuberculosis and sent him to a sanatorium. In an advanced stage of tuberculosis, Bunyan was released from the crowded sanatorium too soon and returned home. Before he died, he had infected both his wife and child. The Bunyan family, including Bunyan's grandmother, had been living in a dirty, congested tenement house. Grandmother Bunyan had been for twenty years an active carrier of tuberculosis germs. Among those responsible for Bunyan's death were: the landlord who had not altered the living conditions; the first doctor for relying on the stethoscope; the second doctor who, wise enough to use the x-ray, had been negligent in not examining Bunyan's family; the sanatorium officials for having released the patient prematurely; and the government for having allowed a man who was 50% handicapped and a danger to both his family and society to return to his family and his work.

Acting as judge and jury, Bethune indicted all of these and then delivered a list of suggestions, some of them most radical for the time, to prevent such deaths. To inform the general public of the nature of tuberculosis, an extensive publicity campaign was necessary. Medical students should receive more information concerning the disease. Regular x-rays of school children would provide for early detection of tuberculosis. All nurses, nursemaids and food handlers in Montreal should receive thorough physical examinations. All known active tubercular cases should be segregated. Finally, a "half-way house" between sanatoria and industry should be established where partly cured tubercular patients could be sent to work in light industries. These industries would be subsidized and protected by the government, the only agency with the capital and the necessary powers to implement his broad-ranging schemes.

His new and radical views were shared by only a few colleagues, politicians and laymen. Working with George Mooney, who was a Y.M.C.A. secretary in the Montreal suburb of Verdun, Bethune opened a free clinic. Every Saturday at noon, he treated without charge women, children and unemployed men in Mooney's office. The Verdun clinic was almost a political act, Bethune's spontaneous, angry reaction to his own profession and a government indifferent to suffering, but he remained politically conservative. At a Canadian Club luncheon in 1935 Bethune's angry disagreement with a speaker who was praising the Russian medical system became so intense that Mooney had trouble preventing him from openly challenging the speaker during the address. After the meeting, Mooney told Bethune that the only way of judging the speaker's opinions was to go to Soviet Russia to learn for himself.

In August Bethune went to Moscow and Leningrad to attend the International Physiological Congress. The Congress itself, and the presence of the great Russian scientist, Ivan Pavlov, held little attraction for him. He had gone for other reasons as he later explained:

Now I did not go ... to Russia to attend a physiological

congress. I went to Russia for much more important reasons
than that. I went to Russia primarily to look at the Russians,
and secondarily to see what they were doing about eradi-
cating one of the most easily eradicable of all contagious
diseases—tuberculosis.

Bethune visited hospitals and clinics, constantly making
mental notes, questioning, praising, openly criticizing. At
one point he repeatedly challenged a Soviet official's claim
that the regime had eliminated prostitution. Ignoring the
agitated official's statistical arguments, Bethune offered
to escort him to the Moscow streets to prove his point.

After more than three weeks during which he had been
"... swimming in the Neva, walking about unhindered
in the streets, looking into windows, making the rounds
of the picture galleries and markets and shops—a combination of Walter Winchell, Peeping Tom and an Innocent
Abroad," he returned to Montreal. On the night of his
arrival he saw Jean Palardy at a lecture given by Norman
Thomas, the American Socialist leader. He told Palardy
he had seen "extraordinary things" and, though he had
thought it necessary to confound some boastful Soviet doctors, he came away deeply impressed with their system
of hospitalization, welfare and social medicine. Visitors to
the Soviet Union were rare in the mid-thirties and their
observations and opinions were eagerly heard, especially
if they confirmed existing Canadian prejudices. As he
described his reactions to the U.S.S.R., he was irritated
by the hostility of anti-Communist feeling he met and this
tended to exaggerate his positive responses to the trip.

In December, 1935, the Montreal Medico-Chirurgical
Society invited the four doctors who had attended the Con-
gress to reveal their impressions at a Society meeting.
Bethune spoke last deliberately:

I made up my mind to take the opposite position to those
held by the others, as I felt fairly sure they would be unani-
mous. If they deprecated Russia I would praise her, and
if they praised, I would diminish her. This would not be

done in a spirit of pure perversity but from a concern for truth, which appears to me to consist not infrequently in the conjunction of apparently irreconcilable aspects of reality. Whatever one says about Russia is true—relatively true—and not in any absolute terms, of course.

After a brief and witty comparison of Soviet Russia and Lewis Carroll's "Wonderland," he suggested the possible contrasting observations and opinions that visitors to the U.S.S.R. might reach:

Isadora Duncan, in the story of her life, describes her confinement: "There I lay, a fountain spouting blood, milk and tears." What would a person think, watching for the first time a woman in labour and not knowing what was occurring to her? Would he not be appalled at the blood, the agony, the apparent cruelty of the attendants, the whole revolting technique of delivery? He would cry, "Stop this, do something, help, police, murder!" Then tell him that what he was seeing was a new life being brought into the world, that the pain would pass, that the agony and the ugliness were necessary and always would be necessary to birth. Knowing this, then what could he say truthfully about this woman as she lies there? Is she not ugly?—yes; is she not beautiful?—yes; is she not pitiful, ludicrous, grotesque and absurd?—yes; and *all* these things would be true.

Now Russia is going through her rebirth, and the midwives and obstetricians have been so busy keeping the precious baby alive that they haven't got around as yet to cleaning up the mess. And it is this mess, the ugly uncomfortable and sometimes stupid mess, which affronts the eyes and elevates the noses of those timid male and female virgins suffering from frigid sterility of the soul . . . who lack the imagination to see behind the blood the significance of birth. Creation is not and never has been a genteel gesture. It is rude, violent and revolutionary. But to those courageous hearts who believe in the unlimited future of man, his divine destiny which lies in his own hands to make of it what he will, Russia presents today the most exciting spectacle of the evolutionary, emergent and heroic spirit of man which has appeared on this earth since the Renaissance.

> To deny this is to deny your faith in man, and that is
> the unforgivable sin, the final apostasy.

The speech caused considerable comment in the medical
community but was not publicized beyond that. To those
few who could claim to know Bethune, his praise of the
Soviet Union was not surprising, and to some it was even
predictable. But to others this was Bethune's final apostasy.
He was outspoken professionally; he was a rebel socially;
he had now assumed a highly unpopular stand politically.
Clearly, "he didn't fit in here."

Even before his December speech, he had reached a
basic decision on the organization of medical care in
Canada. Compared to the Soviet Union the Canadian system was incredibly backward. Inspired by the Soviet example, he began work on a plan to force Canadian governments on all levels to adopt socialized medicine. In the
fall of 1935 he brought together in his apartment a group
of doctors, nurses, dentists, social workers and laymen
interested in the problems of health care. With Bethune
acting as chairman they decided to lay out a detailed plan
for a policy of socialized medicine. Each of the members
of what became known as the Montreal Group for the
Security of the People's Health was given a research task.
The first purpose was to analyse the organization of medical
care in each of the major European nations and to compare
them with those of Canada and the United States.

Throughout the winter and spring of 1936 the group
held meetings to present reports and argue their many
points of view. Bethune guided the group through their
deliberations, built up research material, and made
speeches urging government action. In Memphis, Tennes-
see, speaking on developments in chest surgery to the Mid-
South Post-Graduate Medical Assembly, he concluded with
a dramatic presentation of the case for state medicine:

> The contest in the world today is between two kinds of
> men: those who believe in the old jungle individualism,
> and those who believe in co-operative efforts for the secur-
> ing of a better life for all.

Let us abandon our isolation and grasp the realities of the present economic crisis. The world is changing beneath our very eyes and already the bark of Aesculapius is beginning to feel beneath its keel the great surge and movement of the rising world tide which is sweeping on, obliterating old landscapes and old scenes, not to be turned back by the King Canute of the American Medical Association.

Dr. Duane Carr, who had invited Bethune to Memphis, said of the speech: "[It] caused quite a sensation. This was ... one of the most conservative areas in the United States, a fact which he readily sensed and it was my impression that he laid it on somewhat thicker than he actually felt because he was thoroughly enjoying the reaction of his audience."

Many doctors were concerned by the effects of the Depression on the quality of medical care in Canada, though very few were willing to endorse Bethune's radical solutions to the problems. In April, 1936, the Montreal Medico-Chirurgical Society invited Bethune to make his case for socialized medicine at its monthly meeting. He began by arguing that the question of medical care was ethical and moral and related directly to social and political as well as medical economics. The practice of medicine in Canada was determined by capitalism, a system facing a serious economic crisis, a "deadly disease requiring systematic treatment" but "those palliative measures as suggested by most of our political quacks are aspirin tablets for a syphilitic headache. They may relieve, they will never cure." Using data provided by various recent American studies he argued that under existing conditions a surprisingly large percentage of people were receiving virtually no medical care whatsoever. At the same time, on the basis of the fee-for-service basis which he described as "morally disturbing," many doctors were being inadequately paid because most people were unable to meet their medical bills.

He then outlined his solutions to the problems. Urging that the system must be changed, that fee-for-service, private charity and philanthropic institutions as means of improving social welfare were inequitable, degrading, inefficient and anachronistic, he demanded that the government assume the responsibility of providing health care for all citizens:

> Socialized medicine and the abolition or restriction of private practice would appear to be the realistic solution of the problem. Let us take the profit, the private economic profit out of Medicine, and purify our profession of rapacious individualism. Let us make it disgraceful to enrich ourselves at the expense of the miseries of our fellow men. Let us organize ourselves so that we can no longer be exploited by our politicians. Let us redefine medical ethics—not as a code of professional etiquette between doctors, but as a code of fundamental morality and justice between Medicine and the people.

He urged the unification of all medical and social workers into a "great army... to make a collectivized attack on disease." By organizing in this manner, through the exercise of democratic self-government among themselves, all health workers could present a plan for socialized medicine to government. Under the plan, government could then abolish all forms of charitable organizations. All health care would be state-controlled, managed by health workers paid by the state.

The philosophic basis of Bethune's argument had already been adopted by the Montreal Group for the Security of the People's Health. Three months later they prepared a detailed working plan of a system of state medical care. Their proposal suggested several experimental plans which under proper management would be checked against each other. On the basis of the results at the end of the trial period, a plan for the entire province could be formulated. The four trial plans were:

1. A system of municipal medicine. One Montreal hospital would be selected for which all staff members would be salaried. All costs and salaries would be met by municipal taxes and provincial grants. The hospital would

be subjected to close scrutiny to determine costs in order that it be placed on a sound actuarial basis.

2. Compulsory health insurance. An entire community would pay health insurance to determine actual costs and the ability of the community to meet the costs.
3. Voluntary health insurance. This would be offered in one community of five to ten thousand people.
4. Care of the unemployed. This would be adopted only on a fee-for-service basis throughout the Province of Quebec to be financed from taxation.

These proposals were included in a 3,500 word report summarizing the committee's findings after more than six months' examination of existing health plans in various countries. Essentially the report endorsed the concept of socialized medicine and suggested that by a systematic application of their four proposals a viable plan suitable to Canadian conditions could be formulated. In July, 1936, on the eve of a Quebec provincial election, the report was presented to Premier Godbout, Maurice Duplessis, the leader of the opposition, and to each of the more than fifty candidates in Montreal. Copies had already been sent to all medical, dental and nursing societies, to social and charitable agencies and to the religious authorities in Montreal.

The reaction of the medical profession, the political parties and the public was bitterly disappointing to Bethune. The months of reading, lengthy meetings at his apartment, personal discussions, speeches and powerful emotional effort all ended in futility. Generally the medical people were hostile. They feared government and they believed they would lose their rights as individuals. In the light of future developments, none of these plans was radical; in 1936, they all were. Neither the politicians nor the public was willing to accept anything so heavily state-controlled. Fear of Russian communism doomed the group and Bethune's hopes. The failure of the proposal to elicit more than isolated voices of support, and the indifference and hostility in many quarters upset him. But he was not shocked, only saddened. He had foreseen the probable result even as he threw all his physical, intellectual and emotional resources into the campaign. Far better than most men, he could assess difficulty, face risk, and survive temporary defeat if the cause was urgent.

The rejection by the medical profession was the hardest to bear. Although he understood their distaste for his social behaviour, he could not accept their apparent inability to separate the man from his medical and political concepts. Doctors outside the operating or consultation room seemed to lose the perspective that made them successful within their own professional environment. Many of them were afraid of the steps that he saw were necessary to improve the physical well-being of the public. Others were unconcerned, content to restrict their interests to the technical side of their speciality.

He had felt this strongly when he pleaded with his profession to take the steps he believed they knew could eradicate tuberculosis. Too few seemed able or willing to look beyond the immediate. This was no less true when he advocated the adoption of a form of socialized medicine. In his April speech to the Medico-Chirurgical Society he had implored his colleagues to

> ... discuss more often the great problems of our age and not so much the interesting cases; the relationship of Medicine to the State; the duties of the profession to the people; the matrix of economics and sociology in which we exist. Let us recognize that our most important contemporaneous problems are economic and social and not technical and scientific in the narrow sense that we employ those words.

He had always regarded doctors as narrow and lacking interest in cultural pursuits. Now he believed they were guilty of a more damaging charge. Their prime interest appeared to be their own social status, the direct result of their profits from the practice of medicine. Bethune posed a threat to this as the advocate of a scheme that would change radically their independent social and economic position.

The rejection of his plans by his profession was also a great blow to his self-esteem. He was always looking for recognition: "He wanted desperately to be meaningful." Yet he was growing away from his own profession, living on the fringes of society, ostracized and disoriented. He was searching constantly for a means of self-expression that would match his desire to live life significantly and vividly. He found it in Marxist Communism.

Although he had rejected organized Christianity, he still retained the evangelical zeal of his missionary parents. He was deeply aware of this when he wrote, "My father was an evangelist and I come from a race of men ... of passionate convictions ... with ... a vision of truth ...." In all his actions there was ample evidence of "a tremendous impulse to act, to do." In the Communist movement, he found similar characteristics. They too were committed to action and willing to pursue a course of action to completion in a way that appealed to Bethune. He liked as well their commitment to a social and political *tabula rasa* upon which to plan the future. By definition, they opposed tradition and vested interests. Through revolution, the past was to end and the future begin. This was the political equivalent to Bethune's own thinking about some aspects of medicine.

The intellectual basis of Marxism interested him. He had read little Marxist literature, but his adept mind absorbed quickly. Stanley Ryerson, Secretary of the Quebec Communist Party, who gave a series of lectures in late 1935 attended by Bethune, recalls:

I remember his asking "What shall I read?" and [my] saying, "Start with the *Communist Manifesto* and Engel's *Socialism: Scientific and Utopian* and Lenin's *The State and Revolution*. I think that he read most of the basic works, but I think that he never had the time nor the opportunity to read more fully ... to really make a study of questions of theory ... but he was theoretically very active .... Questions of reality and experience would detonate big questions in his mind which he would instantly wrestle with .... He had a terrific instaneity of insight and a cast of mind that led him quickly to [the] interaction between practical [and theoretical] things.

His first direct contact with the Canadian Communist Party came on his return from the Soviet Union. Louis Kon, a naturalized Canadian of Russian birth who had formed an organization called "The Friends of the Soviet Union", was attracted by Bethune's descriptions of his recent trip. After an introductory meeting during which Kon loaned Bethune a book, *Moscow Dialogues,* he invited Bethune to become chairman of the organization. His first reactions were revealed in a letter to Marian Scott:

> ... It would appear that Sir Andrew MacPhail had spoken about or recommended me. Why I can't say for since my trip, my expressions have not been entirely complimentary in some quarters (depending of course on my audience!—enthusiastic to the reactionaries, minimizing to the radical).
>
> Now, it is rather a question to me whether or not I can conscientiously take such a position. I explained my attitude frankly to Mr. K_____ saying definitely that though in theory I am entirely in agreement with the ideology of this modern religion, yet I was disturbed and rather deeply disturbed in some of its aspects in practice. In short, that I did not believe that communism as practised in Russia today was a suitable technique for the Anglo-Saxons (predominantly Anglo-Saxon, at heart) of this country ... but that basically ... I was in deep sympathy with Russia. To my surprise he agreed with me.
>
> I added that I was profoundly distrustful of social democracy and of the C.C.F. in their non-realization of the absolute inevitability of the use of force and force alone as the only true persuader.
>
> Moneyed people will *never* give up money and power until subjugated by physical forces stronger than they possess. Democracy will come again, as it will come again in Russia, only after the people are conditioned, as they are being conditioned, to their new manner of living, but democracy at first is shiftless, careless, ignorant and willful. Only when the course is set can it be permitted to guide the ship.

Well, what shall I do? Do you think I can conscientiously take this job? I don't think I know enough. I feel very ignorant. Yet I feel a tremendous impulse to do, to act. I hate to be thought one of the intelligentsia who talk and talk and talk and believe their words. You feel their hearts are cold and it's only an intellectual conundrum. A game.

Bethune, hospitalized at this time with a severe case of jaundice, took some time to decide. Almost three weeks later he answered Louis Kon:

I am extremely obliged to you for your kindness in lending me "Moscow Dialogues." I am finding it extremely interesting as the philosophy underlying communism had never been explained to my satisfaction . . . .

Now in regard to the other matter of the chairmanship—I will be perfectly frank with you so you will understand my position exactly.

I do not feel able to accept for two reasons. The first is that I am not, as yet, perfectly convinced that communism is the solution to the problem. If I were, I assure you, I should not only accept your offer but would become a member of the Communist party. What stands in the way of my acceptance? This—my strong feeling of individualism—the right of a man to walk alone, if that's his nature—my dislike of crowds and regimentation. Perhaps all these fears are illusionary and do not necessarily conflict with the *practice* of communism, even though they seem to be solved in its theory, but I am afraid. This being so I must read more, think more about this problem. In short, I am not yet ready.

Second, such being the case—to jeopardize the only position—economic and professional—I possess, by even associating with a communistic-leaning association such as yours would be senseless. If I felt as strongly and as purely towards communism as perhaps I should, such jeopardization of my means of livelihood would not be an obstacle in any way. But the ironic and ludicrous picture of a half-hearted convert, reluctantly being burnt at the stake for his half-hearted, feeble convictions, rises in my mind.

So it all hinges on this—I am not ready as yet to throw in my lot with you.

82

But his lot was solitary, and alone he could not act effectively. He continued to study the theoretical basis of Marxism, and in early 1936 began to attend Communist Party meetings.*

In May, 1936, he went to the annual convention of the American Association of Thoracic Surgery bristling with a desire to deflate the complacent and insensitive thoracic surgeons. With him he brought a paper which he had been preparing for several months entitled "Some errors in technique and mistakes in judgement made in the course of 1,000 thoracic surgical operations." He wrote to Dr. Richard Meade, whom he was helping with the programme: "That should startle them!—I'm getting very tired (and envious!) of successful brilliant results [so] I have collected 25 'howlers' of my own & would [want] others to join me at the public confessional for the benefit of the young." His paper did startle and infuriate many. Others were impressed. Dr. Duane Carr, in describing Bethune as "courageous", regarded his motive as wanting "... to help others to avoid the errors which he had made himself. It was most valuable to the younger men who heard the papers and, if they listened, they were better thoracic surgeons for doing so." Bethune, of course, had not committed 1,000 errors but many thoracic surgeons were strongly opposed to publicizing a confession by one of their prominent colleagues, no matter what its purpose, and the paper was never published. His mood at the convention was described by a colleague:

... he had a black shirt on that he obviously hadn't changed

*A number of Communists were interviewed or corresponded with to determine more precisely the date of Bethune's entry. No records were kept, especially after 1937 when the Padlock Law of Quebec authorized searches of homes and other dwellings in order to confiscate all manner of documents. The law was directed against the Communist Party. No one, including Stanley Ryerson, Tim Buck, the national leader, and Sam Carr, the national organizer, could give an exact date. Since he decided as late as October 18, 1935, not to join and was a member upon his arrival in Spain, he joined sometime in 1936. Since he appeared at meetings in early 1936, the assumption follows that his membership began in the spring of that year.

in a month. He had a little handbag which he opened and
showed me. He carried a phone book in it so that when
he checked into a hotel he would have evidence that he
had baggage, although he had none and was travelling
very light. . . . He had trouble getting the car started so
one of the fellows suggested that he might be out of
gas . . . . He went into the hotel and got a coat hanger to
measure the gas because there was no gas meter on the
car. The car had been sitting there in front of the hotel
for three days and hadn't been used since he had arrived
in Rochester . . . . We soon found out by exploring the gas
tank with the coat hanger that Norman had a dry tank.
He had driven up to the hotel and just made it, but that
was Norman's life.

Bethune returned to Montreal in June. As usual he had
gained only temporary satisfaction from his snarling
defiance. Meanwhile he was forced to face the loneliness
of his personal life. Longing for companionship, he had
tried vainly to fill the gap created by the loss of Frances.
He knew many women in Montreal and, according to Dr.
Geddes,

He had an extraordinary attraction to women. They loved
to listen to him talk and they liked to follow him around.
I don't think I ever knew anyone who attracted women
to him more like a magnet than he did. One brilliant woman,
I recall, and a very beautiful woman . . . said, "I saw him
but once and he was the most aggressively male creature
I have ever encountered."

In 1935 he fell deeply in love with a married woman and
for a time he believed that a permanent relationship might
develop. It never did. He wrote to her:

It is pleasant to sit and think that you are near me, close
beside me, only a few streets away. I am very conscious
of your presence and happy because of it—yet sad too,
darling, because of the knowledge that you and I are bound
together, to work out some part of our lives together—for
good or for evil—we seem to be bound.
    Perhaps this is a presumption on my part—but I think

not. And if your glance, your touch, your hands and lips are not mistaken, unreal or misread—you feel it too.

Do you remember the girl in "Farewell To Arms" saying with that mysterious foresight of love "Let us be good to each other. We are to have such a strange life together," and her lover comforts her sad heart as best he may, not hearing or understanding. But she knew the dark paths ahead.

Well, my sweet, I know it too. Let me persuade you to stop now. Go back. Put away this small child of our love you are holding so gently and tenderly in your cupped hands—now, when it can be put away without agony and tears—before it has grown in stature and strength and threatens to destroy all you hold precious in life . . . .

And I say this because I am persuaded there is something fated and doomed and predestined about myself.

But again I think—us. Let us go on into the future together—heads up and with a smile on our lips. If we are true to ourselves, the future might be happy (O I am afraid so afraid for you)—but no real harm or injury can touch us—nothing can come from without to destroy us. This is the way I try to persuade myself and you.

Dare we risk it?

It is because I love you I write like this, so darkly, lest I injure you with my love and do you a harm. Instead of bedecking you with jewels, I load you with chains;

Beth, your sad lover

Madrid is the Centre
of the World

On the morning of July 18, 1936, Madrid radio announced the outbreak of a rebellion among Spanish Army units stationed in the African Protectorate of Morocco. Attempting to reassure loyal listeners, the government announcer cautioned that the revolt "was confined to certain areas of the Protectorate and that no one, absolutely no one, on the mainland has joined such an absurd venture." Far from being an isolated event, the Moroccan insurrection was part of a series of planned uprisings taking place throughout Spain that same day. Within a few days the "absurd venture" had thrust the Spanish people into an intense and bitter war whose ideological overtones soon made it the focus of world interest.

The revolt was led by General Francisco Franco, the Chief of the General Staff, who headed the right-wing Nationalist forces supported by landowners, businessmen, the Catholic hierarchy, and many military leaders. The Republicans, who had won the elections in February of 1936 by forming a Popular Front coalition with the Socialists, Anarchists and Communists, were backed by the Loyalists, comprising intellectuals, agricultural labourers, and the urban working class. At first the coup was a failure.

85

Some army leaders hesitated, then finally reneged. Most air force and naval officers confounded the rebels by remaining loyal. In the two biggest cities, Barcelona and Madrid, the coup failed completely and the conspirators were forced to surrender. During the first confusion, the government hesitated, made changes in the cabinet, and eventually announced the abolition of the army, leaving the country virtually defenceless. Union leaders demanded that the government open the armouries to the masses, and the new Prime Minister finally agreed. The Republic's citizen army began to take shape as the workers seized arms and began to confront the rebels in the streets and in the countryside. Within weeks of the outbreak, German and Italian men and materiel began arriving to help Franco drive back the untrained Loyalists. By September, with 40% of Spain in Nationalist hands, government forces were retreating in every area. By the beginning of November, Madrid itself was under seige.

Events in Spain immediately captured newspaper headlines around the world. Journalists streamed into Madrid and sent back despatches from the shifting front. Initially world opinion tended to favour the Republic, a legally elected government threatened from within by outlaw forces. Support increased when Franco introduced the German and Italian troops, whose terribly efficient use of dive bombers and tanks unmasked the new and savage face of modern warfare.

Even during the early days of the conflict there were those abroad who cheered on Franco's advances. The Spanish Catholic Church, an open enemy of the Republic since its inception, energized its effective propaganda machine to counter much of the liberal opinion in other countries. Spaniards and outsiders alike were horrified by the excesses of vengeance exacted upon the Church within the Loyalist zone. During the first confusing weeks before the Loyalist government was able to exercise full civil and military control, the smouldering antagonism harboured by many Spaniards erupted in the destruction of Churches and the execution of priests. Heedless of the numerous and officially authorized atrocities in the Nationalist zones, the Catholic Church encouraged the belief that Franco was at the head of a modern crusade that, according to the Archbishop of Toledo, would crush "the modern monster, Marxism, or Communism, the seven-headed hydra, symbol of all heresies."

But it was the political complexion of Loyalist Spain that most influenced non-Catholics as well as Catholics. In early September, with tensions rising and defeatism threatening, Largo Caballero, the Socialist leader, was installed as Prime Minister. In an effort to integrate support from the various elements of the Popular Front, he invited both Communist and Anarchist participation in his cabinet. Two Communists entered the cabinet, the first in any Western democratic government. In November the Anarchists followed.

The growing conservative belief that power in Madrid was in the hands of "the seven-headed hydra" was strengthened immeasurably with the arrival of Russian tanks and airplanes in October. Soviet military aid was minimal, and, to the Loyalists, despairingly irregular by contrast to the aid provided the Nationalists by Germany and Italy. Nevertheless, to many observers, this represented the ultimate proof that Loyalist Spain had become an instrument of International Communism.

Throughout the late summer and early autumn of 1936 the Civil War held world attention. Spain became the most important political fact of the 1930's. Many people believed a decisive battle was being waged between Communism and Fascism, the two predominant ideological forces to have developed since World War One. The Spanish magnet attracted not only journalists but writers, intellectuals, artists, photographers, members of parliament and the merely curious who reported their observations in newspapers, novels, articles, newsreels and speeches to an absorbed world.

Among those who went to Spain to aid the government were almost 40,000 men and women who had chosen to make history rather than report it. They came from more than sixty countries. Perhaps half were Communists who

answered the call of the Comintern to place themselves
at the disposal of the Loyalist government. Many, however,
were idealists, socialists and liberals frustrated by the
Depression, eager to do something tangible, and united
by a common conviction that fascism represented the most
serious threat to world peace. In Spain they gathered in
national units to form the romantic and militarily effective
International Brigades. Among them were 1,200 Canadians of the Mackenzie-Papineau Battalion. Many who
were no less committed to the anti-fascist cause chose to
contribute in other ways. Throughout Europe and North
America committees were hastily formed to send medical
aid and relief supplies to the beleaguered Republic. The
political composition of these various committees was
similar to that of the Brigades.

The Canadian relief committee began in early October
at the initiative of A.A. McLeod, chairman of the Canadian
branch of the League Against War and Fascism. McLeod
and Tim Buck, Secretary of the Communist Party of
Canada, were in Brussels to attend the Universal Peace
Conference during the first week of September. Following
the Conference, they went to Madrid to determine how
they could be useful to the Republic. Back in Canada they
began to lay the groundwork for the Committee to Aid
Spanish Democracy.

When the Civil War began, Bethune and members of
the Montreal Group for the Security of the People's Health
were making final arrangements for the printing of their
manifesto in support of socialized medicine. Reports of
the negative reactions of both doctors and politicians came
to Bethune at the same time as the news from Spain grew
worse. In August, as his mood became blacker, he openly
expressed contempt for his own profession and the reac-
tionary forces under Franco. While most of his colleagues
at Sacré Coeur were aware of his feelings and some shared
them, the Catholic hospital authorities were less understanding, and the atmosphere grew tense. His concern with
events in Spain moved him to write a poem called "Red
Moon":

And this same pallid moon tonight,
Which rides so quietly, clear and high,
The mirror of our pale and troubled gaze
Raised to a cool Canadian sky,

Above the shattered Spanish tops
Last night rose low and wild and red,
Reflecting back from her illumined shield
The blood bespattered faces of the dead.

To that pale disc we raise our clenched fists,
And to those nameless dead our vows renew,
"Comrades, who fought for freedom and the future world,
Who died for us, we will remember you."

In September, after a lengthy and emotional discussion concerning events in Spain, he asked a friend, "I'd like to go over there. What do you think? Can you lend me $200?" When the friend was unable to raise the money, Bethune decided to offer his services to the Red Cross. To his angry surprise he received a reply from the National Commissioner which said, in part, "The Canadian Red Cross Society is not raising a Unit for Service in Spain and has not, I think, any intention whatever of doing so."

Shortly after learning of the Red Cross decision he read in the *New Commonwealth,* the C.C.F. weekly newspaper, an article outlining the formation of the Spanish Hospital and Medical Aid Committee. The Toronto-based organization was planning to send personnel and supplies to Madrid to establish a hospital there. Bethune immediately wired the editor, Graham Spry, to offer his services and to announce that he would arrive in Toronto the following day to discuss the details. Spry was both delighted and alarmed. The Spanish Hospital and Medical Aid Committee was an imaginary creation he had hoped would stir interest in the plight of the Republic and eventually become a reality. When Bethune arrived the following day, Spry confessed that there was neither an organization nor money to send him to Spain.

Bethune was dismayed for only a moment. He and Spry

soon were talking enthusiastically of actually founding the Spanish Hospital and Medical Aid Committee. Spry promised to contact leading anti-fascists, among them A.A. McLeod, who had just returned from Spain. Their only asset was the return portion of a steamship ticket a student had given Spry for Bethune. The Committee to Aid Spanish Democracy (C.A.S.D.), as the group was now called, began to take shape. They enlisted support from all sectors of anti-fascist opinion.* Two Protestant ministers were invited to head the executive: Reverend Salem Bland as Honorary Chairman, and, as Chairman, Reverend Benjamin Spence, a well-known Torontonian and veteran Prohibitionist. McLeod, Buck, Spry and Dr. Rose Henderson, a liberal, were vice-chairmen. During its three-year history, the C.A.S.D. raised thousands of dollars and set up affiliated committees throughout Canada. The Communist party was careful to avoid appearing in a dominant role but through the forceful personalities of McLeod and Buck and the total commitment of other Party members who were always willing to do the hack work, Communist influence was out of proportion to the number of its members involved.

After his first meeting with Spry, Bethune had ample time to consider his future. Montreal had brought him moments of pleasure but it also had convinced him that he was out of step with his own profession. Although he had enjoyed the company of some Montrealers, his personal life was lonely, he was a political alien, deeply anti-fascist, and a member of the Communist Party of Canada. He told a friend, "It is in Spain that the real issues of our time are going to be fought out. It is there that democracy will either die or survive." On October 17 he resigned

*The Committee to Aid Spanish Democracy was the sole instance in Canada of the Popular Front concept whereby all left-wing factions would temporarily unite for a specific common cause. Neither before the Civil War nor after was there any cooperation between Canadian Socialists and Communists. For this reason there were C.C.F. members who refused to work for the C.A.S.D. since any agreement with Communists invited "the kiss of death."

from his position at the Veterans' Hospital, and his letter of resignation from Sacré Coeur was sent several days later. On October 24 he boarded a ship at Quebec City armed with a quantity of medical supplies, American Express money orders and a letter of introduction to Prime Minister Caballero. His last words before leaving were, "Whether or not Madrid falls before the invading forces, I will complete my mission."

As the S.S. Empress of Britain carried Bethune across the North Atlantic, four columns of Nationalist troops were moving inexorably toward Madrid, driving before them the retreating Republican forces. Intensive bombing of the capital began on the night of October 29, partly as a German experiment to discover the effects of modern aerial bombardment on a crowded civilian population. On November 7, as the Caballero government and most embassy staffs were leaving for Valencia, newspaper correspondents prepared their descriptions of the fall of Madrid. At dawn on November 8, under cover of a heavy bombardment, 20,000 disciplined and well-armed Moroccan troops and legionnaires moved into the suburbs of Madrid in the sector known as University City. Ranged against them was a hastily formed defence comprising the famous Communist Fifth Regiment, militiamen, workers, and the first units of the International Brigades. So badly equipped that the worker soldiers waited behind barricades to recover the guns of dead comrades in order to replace them in the line, the Loyalist troops were fired with an incredible zeal. Day after day, under bombing so intense that the defenders seemed to be "treading blood and breathing sparks," the Madrileños survived the first aerial saturation attack. After nearly three weeks Franco revised his strategy and proposed a flanking movement to surround the city. Madrid was given a breathing spell.

Bethune arrived in Madrid on November 3 and took a room in the Gran Via Hotel, a popular location for many of the foreign correspondents and observers. Here- he planned to meet Henning Sorensen, a Montrealer who had agreed to represent the *New Commonwealth* and a Danish labour newspaper in Spain. Before Sorensen left Canada in September, Spry had also asked him to report on medical conditions for the proposed Committee. After it had grown into the more substantial Committee to Aid Spanish Democracy, Canadian officials wired Sorensen asking him to meet Bethune in Madrid.

While he waited for Sorensen on his second day in Madrid, Bethune was eyed suspiciously by a militiaman in a café. As he entered the hotel lobby he was stopped by the pursuing militiaman who began to talk excitedly in Spanish. Bethune turned to a hotel clerk for help. After questioning the man, the clerk explained that because Bethune was well-dressed, wore a moustache and had used the word "fascist" in the café, the militiaman had become convinced he was a spy. Bethune laughed and went up to his room. Minutes later he answered the door to find five armed guards and a police inspector who demanded his identification. After examining Bethune's passport and a safe conduct issued by the Spanish Embassy in Paris, they left. Another knock at the door announced Henning Sorensen. They exchanged greetings and Bethune handed Sorensen a letter for him from Canada. Suddenly the door was opened by the police inspector who bolted into the room, grabbed the letter from Sorensen and began to read it. The salutation began with "Darling." The inspector's face reddened as he read on. Embarrassed and angry, he abruptly assured the confused militiaman that neither Bethune nor Sorensen were enemies of the Republic.

The incident was not unusual in the tense atmosphere prevailing during the battle of Madrid. Fifth columnists were everywhere and no one was above suspicion. Nor was the militiaman's concern unnatural. Sorensen's first impressions of Bethune were that he was "a very dapper looking fellow, very well-dressed, snappy hat on his head and a little moustache . . . . He looked more like a police officer on leave than anything else." Bethune shaved off his moustache immediately.

Sorensen was multilingual and a great help to him during his stay in Spain. Bethune had arrived with medical supplies, money and his skills as a surgeon. He tried to find out at once how to use them effectively. After Sorensen brought him up to date on recent events in the war, he agreed to escort Bethune to the military hospitals, which were still insufficient even though many had been improvised for the war. In the centre of Madrid, just yards away from the Prado Museum, were two luxury hotels, the Palace and the Ritz, which had been converted into military hospitals. After a tour of both Bethune decided that the number of surgeons was adequate and rejected an offer to join a surgical team.

They then went to Albacete, the administrative headquarters of the International Brigades, to determine their medical needs. Units were arriving daily and harried officials were searching frantically to accommodate the troops. When they finally were introduced to the confused French doctor in charge, Bethune decided to get out. "I couldn't work with that bastard—he doesn't know what he's doing," he told Sorensen. It would clearly be too long before adequate organization could produce a role for him. Back in Madrid, he decided to go to Valencia and buy an ambulance for one of the hospitals. On the train he put together a series of thoughts that had been developing for several days. Sorensen recalls: "We were sitting . . . facing each other and we put down this little folding wooden table between us. And Bethune was silent for a little while and he said, 'Henning, I think I've got an idea!' And then he started to tell me this idea of blood transfusion."

On his visits to the military hospitals he had noted the inadequate facilities for blood transfusions and he knew that Madrileños had died because of the blood shortage. Many other doctors deeply troubled by the problem had failed to provide an organized system of supplying blood. It was typical of Bethune that he saw the main problem quickly and found a solution. He also realized that a specific medical service would bring publicity to the Canadian Committee to Aid Spanish Democracy:

. . . unless we were able to offer the government some definite proposal and concrete scheme our efforts would peter out ... by this I mean I would simply go into a hospital as a surgeon and that would be the end of the Canadian Unit as a Unit! Now it seemed better to emulate England and Scotland and establish ourselves as a definite entity. England has the "English Hospital", Scotland has the "Scottish Ambulance."

Bethune was not a man to submerge himself anonymously in a hospital surgical team. If there were an opportunity to achieve the extraordinary, he would seize it, even create it. Just as before he had preached the gospel of socialized medicine, now he wanted to be in charge of a service that could save thousands of lives.

In Valencia he was directed to the offices of the Socorro Rojo Internacional, a relief agency for the families of political prisoners, where he laid out his plans to impressed S.R.I. officials who promised him a laboratory and facilities in Madrid. He assured them that the funds to equip and operate the service would be raised in Canada. Bethune and Sorensen returned to Madrid and flew to Paris on November 21. Sorensen was there to translate for him, but Bethune grew impatient with the linguistic problems and left for London, where he consulted haemotologists and studied medical literature to gain as much knowledge of blood transfusion as he could. His basic idea was extremely simple: he would extract blood from donors, store it in refrigerators and deliver it to hospitals where and when it was needed. For this he required a specially constructed vehicle. Lacking the time to find exactly what he wanted, he bought a Ford station wagon with light wooden panelling which the Spanish doctors later fondly termed *la rubia* (the blonde). Inside, custom-made boxes contained a small refrigerator, a sterilizing unit and an incubator, each of which operated on gasoline or kerosene. Other smaller pieces of equipment included vacuum bottles, blood flasks, direct blood transfusion sets, various surgical instruments, blood serum, hurricane lamps and gas masks—a total of 1,875 separate pieces.

To avoid paying duty on his car and medical supplies, Bethune visited the French Embassy to request a *laissez-*

passer. When Embassy officials assured him that permission could be granted if the Canadian government would guarantee that he was a bona fide physician engaged in humanitarian work, Bethune turned to Vincent Massey, the Canadian High Commissioner in London. Massey telegrammed the Canadian Department of External Affairs for advice. The following report was handed to the Minister:

> ... Dr. Bethune's medical mission to Madrid was despatched by the "Committee to Aid Spanish Democracy", 73 Adelaide St. West, Toronto. This is understood to be a Communist organization under the chairmanship of the Reverend Benjamin Spence. And it has been said that Tim Buck is associated with it in some way.

The following day, Massey sent a second telegram, stating that Sorensen would accompany Bethune. In October, Sorensen had introduced himself at the British Embassy in Madrid as the representative of Spry's Spanish Hospital and Medical Aid Committee. The British Foreign Office made inquiries at External Affairs, who in turn contacted Spry. Spry confirmed that Sorensen was a journalist and that his committee, no longer in existence, had merged with the Spence Committee.

The connection of Sorensen and Bethune with the suspect Committee to Aid Spanish Democracy was sufficient to implicate both. The official conducting the investigation sent a memo to the Under Secretary of External Affairs: "I think this changes the complexion of the request. Sorensen is not a medical man but a journalist and a Danish subject, and—it would appear from the earlier correspondence—is likely to have political activities in mind." Later that day High Commissioner Massey received the following telegram from the Minister of External Affairs:

> While Government has full sympathy with any efforts to relieve sufferers on either side of present Spanish conflict, it would not be possible in view of what appears to be the political complexion of this mission as indicated by your

second telegram and by other circumstances to sponsor it by making a formal request such as indicated.

After Massey refused his initial request, the determined Bethune pressed harder and finally obtained a letter of introduction from Lester B. Pearson, at that time a First Secretary in the Department of External Affairs attached to the High Commissioner's Office in London. The letter did not convince the French to issue a *laissez-passer* and Bethune was forced to pay a heavy duty. His fury over the incident remained with him a long time, and when he returned to Canada, he did not hesitate to tell the story in public.

Bethune, Sorensen and Hazen Sise, a young architect from Montreal they had met in London, arrived in Madrid on December 12 and quickly established themselves in a fifteen-room apartment just beneath the central offices of the Socorro Rojo Internacional. Located at 36 Principe de Vergara in north-central Madrid, an upper middle-class area, the apartment seldom suffered from Nationalist bombers, who preferred to terrorize the working-class sectors. Bethune and his staff spent the first few days arranging their equipment and forming a compact laboratory and hospital. The unit, which Bethune named the "Servicio Canadiense de Transfusion de Sangre," included Sorensen as Liaison Officer, Sise as driver and general utility man and Celia Greenspan, an American whose husband was a correspondent for the left-wing American periodical, *New Masses,* as laboratory technician. The Spanish personnel consisted of two doctors and four office workers.

Theirs was not the first transfusion service in Spain. On the same day the revolt began, Dr. Gustavo Pittaluga, Professor of Haematology and Parasitology at the University of Madrid, summoned two of his former students who were interning at the university hospital. Turning over all his transfusion equipment to them, he asked them to begin a transfusion service in the Faculty of Medicine which later became the Republican Army Transfusion Service for the Madrid Front. When the Sanidad Militar (Army Medical Service) learned of Bethune's plans, they agreed to place him in charge of the Madrid Service with the rank of major and install his two doctors and the students under him as captains. The Servicio Canadiense was to assume responsibility for the Madrid Front and the Central sector south of Madrid. The Canadians agreed to supply all equipment and pay the salaries of the employees. Four registered nurses were soon added to the staff. In Barcelona, another service was begun by Dr. Frederic Duran Jorda for the Aragon Front.

In the middle of December the Servicio Canadiense began to function. The first stage was the collection of blood. Heeding the appeal made by radio and newspaper, hundreds of Madrileños appeared at 36 Principe de Vergara during the first week of its operation. A detailed medical record was made of each volunteer and a sample of blood was taken. Provided that he was free from disease and possessed the desired type, a volunteer could be called in every three weeks to donate 500 c.c. of blood. Each donor received a cup of coffee and a certificate to permit him to purchase extra food. Some of the first donors were fascists who were disappointed when they failed to receive some identifiable badge to protect them. By the end of the month, more than 1,000 donors were listed, and blood was being collected at the rate of a gallon per day. The second stage was more difficult. Each 500 c.c. of bottled blood containing the donor's name and the date of extraction was placed in a refrigerator set at a temperature of 1° C. Before the blood was refrigerated, a sodium citrate solution was added to prevent clotting. Bethune was sure blood could be stored up to three weeks but he knew that only experience would determine this.

The third stage was distribution. In December and January Bethune's unit concentrated on supplying almost sixty hospitals in Madrid. When blood was needed, Bethune or one of the doctors would take the bottles and transfer them to heated vacuum bottles. The blood was rushed to the hospital in a knapsack. Bethune described this work:

Our night work is very eerie! We get a phone call for blood. Snatch up a packed bag ... and with our armed guard off we go through the absolutely pitch dark streets and the guns and machine guns and rifle shots sound ... as if they were in the next block, although they are really half a mile away. Without lights we drive. Stop at the hospital and with a searchlight in our hands find our way into the cellar. All the operating rooms in the hospitals have been moved into the basement to avoid falling shrapnel, bricks and stones coming through the operating room ceiling.

After the patient was tested to determine his blood type, the transfusion began:

The man is usually as white as ... paper, mostly shocked, with an imperceptible pulse. He may be exsanguinated also and not so much shocked, but usually is both shocked and exsanguinated. We now inject novocaine over the vein in the bend of the elbow, cut down and find the vein and insert a small glass cannula, then run the blood in. The change in most cases is spectacular. We give him always 500 c.c. of preserved blood and sometimes more and follow it up with saline or 5% glucose solution. The pulse can now be felt and his pale lips have some colour.

When the pressure on Madrid eased slightly in December and January, the Servicio Canadiense averaged three transfusions daily. During the battles of Jarama, Malaga and Guadalajara in February and March, when the service was extended outside the capital, as many as 100 transfusions were given in a single day.

Even before the unit was operating efficiently, Bethune's eyes were searching for more difficult tasks. He had repeatedly insisted that transfusions were needed at the front, and he wrote to Spence:

Transfusion work should be given in Casualty Clearing Stations when they come out of the operating room of the first hospital behind the lines and *before* they are sent back to the rear hospitals. But as Madrid is the front line, our work is mostly here although we go out 25 kilometers to other parts of the line.

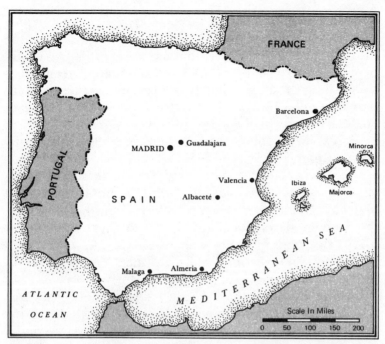

As Franco's strategy changed and Madrid became only a part of the shifting front line, Bethune demanded that the Servicio Canadiense extend its operations to the several fronts. While the Sanidad Militar continued to consider his proposal he went to Marseilles with Sorensen to buy a Renault truck large enough to contain his ever-increasing supply of equipment. Upon his return the Sanidad Militar agreed to extend the operations of the Servicio Canadiense. Blood would be collected in Barcelona by Dr. Duran Jorda and taken to Valencia. Here Bethune would organize a distribution centre for ten front-line hospitals.

Bethune, accompanied by Sise and T.C. Worseley, an English writer, drove the two and one-half ton Renault to Barcelona. While a refrigerator and generator were being installed in the truck, the three men visited Duran Jorda's Transfusion Service. Bethune found the Barcelona Service superior to his own because Duran Jorda, with his more sophisticated equipment, could pool blood in a highly efficient manner, whereas Bethune was forced to use individual bottles. At Barcelona he decided to travel south to Malaga on the Mediterranean coast, where a Nationalist attack had begun January 17, 1937. His purpose was twofold. Blood would certainly be needed by the Republican force of 40,000 militiamen, and the trip would provide an excellent test of the preservation techniques over a long distance. They drove south to Almeria, more than 100 miles northeast of Malaga, arriving on February 10. Malaga, a town of 100,000 inhabitants, was under attack by mechanized Italian and Nationalist units. Shelled by two German cruisers and bombed daily beginning February 3, the civilian population followed orders to evacuate on February 6. They left for Almeria along the coastal highway. While men, women and children fled in terror, the military defence collapsed behind them. Nationalist troops swarmed into the defenceless city, and tanks, supported by aircraft, raced ahead to massacre the tail end of the human column stretching to Almeria.

Despite warnings that Malaga had fallen and that Nationalist troops were advancing, Bethune decided to drive on. Several miles out of Almeria they met the first survivors struggling along the road. As they continued, the procession grew thicker. People begged transportation. Unable to tolerate the distress of the shoeless, hungry and sick women and children, he began to ferry them back to Almeria. For three days and nights, working in shifts, the three men carried their human cargo:

> ... the farther we went the more pitiful the sights became. Thousands of children—we counted five thousand under ten years of age—and at least one thousand of them barefoot and many of them clad only in a single garment. They were slung over their mother's shoulders or clung to her hands. Here a father staggered along with two children of one and two years of age on his back in addition to carrying pots and pans or some treasured possession. The incessant stream of people became so dense we could barely force the car through them.
>
> ... it was difficult to choose which to take. Our car was besieged by a mob of frantic mothers and fathers who with tired outstretched arms held up to us their children, their eyes and faces swollen and congested by four days of sun and dust.

"Take this one." "See this child." "This one is wounded." Children with bloodstained rags wrapped around their arms and legs, children without shoes, their feet swollen to twice their size crying helplessly from pain, hunger and fatigue. Two hundred kilometers of misery. Imagine four days and four nights, hiding by day in the hills as the fascist barbarians pursued them by plane, walking by night packed in a solid stream of men, women, children, mules, donkeys, goats, crying out the names of their separated relatives lost in the mob. How could we choose between taking a child dying of dysentery or a mother silently watching us with great sunken eyes carrying against her open breast her child born on the road two days ago. She had stopped walking for ten hours only. Here was a woman of sixty unable to stagger another step, her gigantic swollen legs with their open varicose ulcers bleeding into her cut linen sandals. Many old people simply gave up the struggle, lay down by the side of the road and waited for death.

We first decided to take only children and mothers. Then the separation between father and child, husband and wife became too cruel to bear. We finished by transporting families with the largest number of young children and the solitary children of which there were hundreds without parents.

And now comes the final barbarism .... On the evening of the 12th when the little seaport of Almeria was completely filled with refugees, its population swollen to double its size, when forty thousand exhausted people had reached a haven of what they thought was safety, we were heavily bombed by German and Italian fascist airplanes. The siren alarm sounded thirty seconds before the first bomb fell. These planes made no effort to hit the government battleship in the harbour or bomb the barracks. They deliberately dropped ten great bombs in the very center of the town where on the main street were sleeping, huddled together on the pavement so closely that a car could pass only with difficulty, the exhausted refugees. After the planes had passed I picked up in my arms three dead children from the pavement in front of the Provincial Committee for the Evacuation of Refugees where they had been standing in a great queue waiting for a cupful of preserved milk and a handful of dry bread, the only food some of them had for days. The street was a shambles of the dead and dying, lit only by the orange glare of burning buildings. In the darkness the moans of the wounded children, shrieks of agonized mothers, the curses of the men rose in a massed cry higher and higher to a pitch of intolerable intensity. One's body felt as heavy as the dead themselves, but empty and hollow, and in one's brain burned a bright flame of hate. That night were murdered fifty civilians and an additional fifty were wounded. There were two soldiers killed.

His anger had been growing for months. From Almeria Bethune returned to Madrid where he threw himself completely into the work of the transfusion service and helped expand it greatly. He described the reorganization in a letter:

We have succeeded in unifying all remaining transfusion units under us. We are serving 100 hospitals and casualty clearing stations in the front lines of Madrid and 100 kilometers from the front of the Sector de Centro. The new name of the Canadian Medical Unit is Instituto Hispano-Canadiense de Transfusion de Sangre. We now have a staff of 25 composed of a haemotologist, bacteriologist, five Spanish doctors, three assistants, six nurses, four technicians, chauffeurs and servants . . . . We collected and gave 10 gallons of blood during January. Expect to increase this to 25 gallons during this month.

This is the first unified blood transfusion service in army and medical history. Plans are well under way to supply the entire Spanish anti-fascist army with preserved blood. Your institute is now operating on a 1,000 kilometer front.

I must leave for Paris immediately to buy 50 additional transfusion apparatuses . . . . The Madrid Defence Junta has given us two new cars. We now have five cars operating here day and night in this sector . . . . Madrid is the centre of gravity of the world. All are well and happy. *No Pasaran!* (They shall not Pass). Salud, Camaradas and Compañeros.

The work was steadily increasing, and he was exhausted. Sorensen describes the effect of the war on Bethune:

He was up early in the morning fresh as a daisy . . . but every afternoon, if he had a chance, he'd go to bed for an hour and sleep solidly. I have seen him go to sleep on the platform in a railway station . . . solidly asleep . . . and then get [up] refreshed . . . . Sometimes fatigue would come over him . . . suddenly . . . and he looked twenty years older.

Bethune went to Paris to purchase more equipment and unwind by enjoying some of the pleasures he had known before going to Spain. After obtaining the supplies, he met a Canadian reporter there and together they went to the championship tennis matches before a riotous night on the town.

He returned to Madrid at the beginning of March. On March 8 Franco initiated a new offensive against the city, this one from the north-east near the town of Guadalajara. Envisioned by Mussolini as a demonstration of Italian military prowess, the battle of Guadalajara instead became the first significant Republican victory of the war. Herbert Matthews, the New York *Times* correspondent, overenthusiastically compared it to Napoleon's defeat at Bailen. During the battle, Bethune and Sorensen were delivering blood to a front-line hospital. Bethune was at the wheel. After leaving their cargo, they drove down the road a quarter-mile from the hospital and came under fire. Bethune stopped the truck and ordered everyone to get out and crawl back to the hospital in the ditches on either side of the road. When they returned to the truck, they found the windshield shattered by a bullet hole on the driver's side. This near contact with death thrilled Bethune, who made a point of driving as near as possible to the front lines:

> He loved getting in danger. He loved the smell of danger . . . . It was always very exciting being with Bethune. You always felt he had a real urge. He needed that adrenalin in the system that comes from a dangerous situation. I got quite frightened with him sometimes, driving blindly into situations. We never knew whether there was a machine gun around the corner, but he would never pause to reconnoitre. He was the cavalry man type.

In the relative safety of Valencia, Bethune himself said,

"I must get back to the front. It is the only place that is real. Life and death are parts of the same picture and if you ignore death the picture is unreal. The front is reality. There is the most beautiful detachment there. Every minute is beautiful because it may be the last and so it is enjoyed to the full."

He wanted to film the transfusion service in action, and suggested the idea to Herbert Kline, a correspondent for the *New Masses*. Kline, a writer, was intrigued but had no movie experience, so he approached a young Hungarian photographer, Geza Karpathi. Together these two amateurs travelled to the front with Bethune and produced one of the classic films to emerge from the Spanish Civil War, *The Heart of Spain*. Under Kline's direction, the documentary film became a tribute to Loyalist resistance and to the efforts of Bethune and his co-workers in the transfusion service.

Bethune deserved the credit. Beginning in early December, 1936, with a small staff and little money, he created in five months a service that supplied blood to every military sector in Spain. He made no specific scientific discovery in the use of preserved blood. His contribution, greater than any discovery that he might have achieved in research, arose from his inflexible determination to take the blood to the wounded near the front. Although Duran Jorda's Barcelona service was scientifically more sophisticated than Bethune's, it was the Instituto's role in the Spanish Civil War to save lives by taking the blood to the wounded, and not the wounded to the blood. Others had conceived the idea before Bethune, but no one had carried it into action. The Spanish rewarded him by granting him the highest military rank held by any foreigner in the medical service—unquestionably his military medical contribution was the greatest in the Spanish Civil War. Perhaps the most significant tribute to him is the fact that mobile blood transfusion units like his own were used by the belligerents in World War II.

The Civil War provided the environment in which his

dominating needs could be satisfied. The act of creating the transfusion service excited him: "A real snappy service can be set up with special badges for donors, stars for each donation . . . it's a beautiful idea . . . and Canadian!" Beyond the creativity was the satisfaction of serving others: "We are well and happy and believe we are doing good. What more can one ask?" In an article describing the delivery of blood to a base hospital near Guadalajara, he clearly revealed the ecstasy of feeling needed: " . . . we feel fine. We feel like a successful salesman who has just placed a big order for goods. This is great! Isn't it grand to be needed, to be wanted?" The chaotic, unpredictable conditions that prevailed during the winter of 1936–37 were exactly those in which he thrived. These were times which demanded the inspirational, rapid decisions he enjoyed making. The element of danger, the fast pace of life, the lack of routine brought out his finest qualities.

Eventually, however, these same elements converged to ignite the impatience that was always ready to burn inside him. In the early months of the war, when the Republic was struggling for its existence and Madrid lay under siege, many of the military and administrative units were operated *ad hoc* by organizations such as the trade unions. Later the Republican government gradually extended its power to control all the various state functions normally belonging to it. During this earlier period Bethune was able to operate as he always liked to—independently. He had justification for this since the funds for the functions of the Service were being raised in Canada by the Spanish Aid Committee. When the Sanidad Militar appointed a control committee of two Spanish doctors in March, 1937 to coordinate the Instituto's activities, Bethune felt constrained and reacted strongly, much as he had in the past, against the enveloping arms of authority. Sise recalls that "he had the temperament to operate in a mobile, almost guerilla-warfare situation, but not the temperament to operate in the rather tighter disciplined army that was marching in the spring and summer of 1937."

Bethune angrily rejected the Spanish attempts to force more controls on him.* Sorensen tried to be a peacemaker while interpreting between Bethune and the Spanish officers. Part of the difficulty resulted from the publicity that as Director of the Instituto he was receiving from the foreign and particularly the North American press. Correspondents were always welcome at 36 Principe de Vergara and their visits were frequent. At times the language barrier isolated the Spaniards from the conversation. But the four doctors who worked directly with Bethune always regarded him as a "gentleman, with a presence commanding much authority."

Bethune's own resentment of authority extended to his relationship with the Spanish Communists. Incidents developed when Bethune would drink too much and reveal his hostility towards any attempt to control him. He did not care about diplomatic courtesies, and his outspoken comments about the family quarrels among the left-wing forces did not endear him to either side. In Malaga, a Communist-Anarchist dispute contributed to the Republican defeat. When Bethune reached Valencia, part of his spleen was directed against "about a million of these anarchist bastards that we will have to put up against the wall and shoot." Louis Huot described Bethune's behaviour in Paris:

> He used to derive the greatest pleasure from staying in the most expensive places ... and ordering ... cham-

*The details of this dispute are difficult to obtain, and much of the evidence is conflicting. For example, it has been impossible to learn the relationship between the Instituto and the Barcelona Service. Bethune stated that the Instituto had supreme command, but no documentation exists to support or refute this claim. Bethune apparently met Duran Jorda only twice. According to Dr. Vicente Goyanes, who worked with him, Bethune directed the blood transfusion units for the entire Republican army, and the Instituto itself continued to function until the end of the war. But the geneticist Dr. Herman J. Muller, later a Nobel Prize winner, who worked briefly with the Instituto, said, "The collapse of the Canadian Blood Transfusion Unit was a result of [the] attacks said to have been made by a Spanish Republican Blood Transfusion Unit that was jealous of the Canadian ... one."

pagne . . . . He would go to places like the Tour d'Argent for dinner . . . and getting chits . . . he would pin all this together and derive great pleasure from the idea of the anguish it would cause when he delivered it.

Herbert Kline said that " . . . he was constantly in trouble with the Communists, and they, like myself, felt that he was not disciplined—that means he wasn't a yes man." According to Sise, his behaviour was the result of "over-work, overtiredness . . . and the inability to suffer fools gladly." Eventually the situation became serious enough that A.A. McLeod and another Canadian Communist official, William Kashtan, came to Spain to investigate. They brought Bethune home for a public speaking tour to raise funds for the Instituto.

On May 18, Bethune left "the centre of gravity of the world." There was no champagne, no sense of exhilaration on this voyage: he travelled steerage to save money, and he was filled with remorse. He told Sise, "I have blotted my copybook." He knew he had done great things in Spain, and he was bitter and resentful that his achievements were clouded in a bureaucratic conflict.

An Empty Homeland

His reception in Toronto on June 14, 1937, blew away the bitterness. Hundreds of people were waiting at Union Station. They shouted and milled about him as he walked to the open car which drove him slowly up University Avenue. Behind him were two marching bands and a parade half a mile long that ended at Queen's Park. Here on the lawn before the Ontario Parliament Buildings he spoke to a crowd of more than 5,000 people.

Two days later he returned to Montreal after an absence of eight months. It was a triumphal return. A crowd of 1,000 greeted him at Windsor Station and carried him shoulder high. That night at the Mount Royal Arena he addressed a capacity audience of 8,000. Speaking without notes, he described wartime conditions, the bravery of the Spanish people and the work of the Instituto. The meeting ended with an appeal for funds, and nearly $2,000 was raised.

The Toronto and Montreal speeches were the first in a series he gave, often twice daily, from the beginning of July to mid-September. Under the auspices of the Committee to Aid Spanish Democracy, he spoke in arenas, union halls, theatres, and churches. Travelling by automobile, airplane and ship he crossed northern Ontario, the Prairies, went south to California, north to British Columbia, back across the Prairies, down to Chicago, through Ontario and Quebec to the Maritimes. The size of his audiences ranged from a mere handful in small towns to several thousand in Winnipeg, Vancouver and Toronto, and by the end of September, he said he had addressed 30,000 people. The amount of the collection varied with the degree of political commitment of his audience. At a meeting in Sudbury in July, 700 people gave $22.40. One week later, a Winnipeg audience of 2,000 donated $1,800. By the end of the third week of July, Bethune announced that $4,500 had been collected. Usually the crowd included unemployed workers, students, intellectuals and the merely curious.

Bethune did not like the tour. He wrote to Frances early in July that "Although the public speaking is not to my liking, I will go through with it." At first, perhaps, he did not enjoy the speaking, but his sense of drama was stirred by the crowds. Long before the end of the tour he became an accomplished speaker. He tried to be direct, to state his case clearly and thoroughly to his Canadian and American audiences. One of the most delicate problems was his political affiliation, which he insisted on revealing. Both Communist and non-Communist Committee members were adamant in refusing him this right. This stung him. On a visit to his friend George Holt, he revealed his frustration at being prevented from admitting he was a Communist: "I am fed up.... I wanted to talk. I wanted to admit that I am a Communist Party member."

The temptation was there at every meeting. In his July 14 speech to the Rotary Club of Sault Ste. Marie, Ontario, he became riled when he was introduced as a man who was lured to Spain by adventure. He immediately corrected the statement by saying, "I did not go to Spain because of any adventurous urge but because of a very definite principle involved in the conflict there." Then he charged that because the Premier of Ontario, Mitchell Hepburn, had used "the military and police forces against the workers' sacred right to strike . . . fascism is raising its head in Ontario." The audience, consisting largely of businessmen, was not amused. The secretary's brief notation in the minutes was: "Dr. Bethune was guest speaker and his talk bordered on Communism."

Before the tour started he was interviewed in his hotel by William Strange, a Toronto journalist, who asked him if he was a Communist. Bethune answered from the bathtub: "Most emphatically I am not. What makes you ask?" When Strange remarked on his use of the clenched-fist salute, Bethune replied:

Look here, let's get this thing straight. You can call me a Socialist if you like. I am a Socialist in the same way that millions of sane people are Socialists. I want to see people getting a square deal and I hate Fascism. The clenched fist is used as a "People's Front" salute. It's used in Spain by everybody who is against the Fascists. That's really all it means—anti-Fascism. Why, Premier Blum of France uses it and he's no Communist. I should describe it as a reply to the raised hand-salute of the fascists.

By the time he reached Winnipeg on July 20, 1937, he refused to play the charade any longer. At a banquet given in his honour at the St. Charles Hotel, he calmly stated "I have the honour to be a Communist." Now that he had removed the uncomfortable mask, his speeches bore the unmistakable characteristics of his political beliefs. Before a packed Legion Hall in Saskatoon he told the crowd:

. . . you can't talk about humanity without speaking of the class struggle. I'm preaching it and the sooner the people realize it, the better. The old form of individualism is gone. The day when a person could open the world like an oyster and eat it has passed. The tentacles of the octopus of monopolistic capitalism are stretching out and the aggression of Japan in China is just one more instance of it.

In most of his speeches he recounted the incident of having

to pay duty on the ambulance because the Canadian government was suspicious of the Spanish Aid Committee: "I asked Ottawa for permission to recommend the use of a Canadian ambulance and I was refused by MacKenzie King, the same man who a little later was photographed shaking hands with the biggest murderer in the world to-day—Hitler."

A generation later there are people who remember him clearly during the speaking tour. A woman who heard him speak in Saskatoon recalls her impressions: "His speech was spellbinding to me . . . he certainly had charisma. . . . He seemed remote and to my youthful eyes rather 'tough.' For those of my generation with my political sentiments he was a hero." A doctor who attended his meeting in Vernon, British Columbia, said:

> He was a very impressive man in his tweedy suit, grey hair, and aggressive mien. . . . I had a dime that I was going to spend on a milkshake after the talk so I gave that, and as a result I was asked to shake his hand. He asked my name, what I was going to be when I grew up, and did I play hockey and eat Okanagan apples. . . . He was a tremendous man in my 14 year old opinion and I have never changed my thinking on him.

A listener remembered his speech in Prince Albert, Saskatchewan:

> Certainly the most lasting impression was the sheer driving force of the man . . . . I have yet to hear another who gave such an irresistible impression of sincerity. But there was another quality . . . a sense of something held under control at the cost of supreme effort. I think it was probably a combination of fatigue and anger; certainly the latter was in evidence when, after a collection box was virtually ignored by the audience, he returned to the platform to remind us that Spain was a rehearsal theatre for what was to come in Europe. At that time it was fortunate for some of us younger ones that he was not recruiting for the International Brigades! By the next morning the influence had

begun to wane, but thirty years later it was still strong enough that my first holiday in Spain suffered somewhat from doubts as to whether I should, in conscience, be there.

In Montreal he went to Sacré Coeur Hospital to visit some of his former patients. A doctor described his reception in the hospital where he had worked for more than four years: "... when the poor sisters saw him in the corridor, they ran away. They were afraid of Norman Bethune. He told me that the Mother Superior was afraid that she would meet the devil if she met him. He was hurt by that." It was hard for him to understand that many people believed God marched with Franco and harder to accept the apathetic attitude to events in Spain he met throughout his tour. Apart from the enthusiastic throngs who were spellbound by his graphic portrayals of the terror, blood and folly of modern war, he realized there were many more who remained indifferent and unconcerned. The closed minds were everywhere. A typical reaction was a letter to the editor published a few days after he had spoken in an Ontario town. What, the writer demanded to know, was the relationship between the battlefields of Spain and the serenity of Northern Ontario?

In the small mining towns of the Canadian Rockies and the big cities of Canada and the United States Bethune repeatedly warned that a world war had already begun in Spain and in China, which had just been invaded by Japan. Only action, immediate and forceful, would stop Hitler and the Japanese. He was reminded that Spain was engaged in a civil war in which Canada and the United States had no right to interfere. To Bethune, national politicians were as blind to international dangers as provincial politicians had been to the necessity for socialized medicine. Nor was his own profession any more enlightened. He spoke to a medical group in the U.S. Northwest and, at one point, his exasperation at the political ignorance of these seemingly educated men overcame his common sense and he flew into a rage. In Halifax, Nova Scotia, a group of local doctors invited him to dinner at a private golf club to hear his description of the techniques used in the blood transfusion service. Many years later his host recalls that "he came home very late and fagged. I was greatly annoyed when one of the doctors phoned me and said, 'Please let it not be known that we were entertaining him.' "

Bethune's alienation was so marked that he could not resume his former career:

Norman came back from Spain knowing that things were washed up . . . because of the same kind of apathy as had washed up the medical care programme. . . . He saw in China a similar struggle going on on a large scale and he identified himself with that. . . . In the mood he was in, he could not have settled down in Montreal to professional practice.

Although he was a committed Marxist himself, he was not prepared for the bitter warfare among Communists, Socialists and Anarchists in the fragmented left wing. Regretting his own conflict with the Communist Party, he was now eager to compensate, to regain the faith they had placed in him.

Spain had toughened him. It was a growing period in which his vision of reality came to maturity. Death, destruction, government bureaucracy, the fragmented Left, and civilian apathy in North America combined to make him more resolute. Fascism was to him a political disease, and, just as he had once resolved to eliminate tuberculosis by preventive measures, he was determined to fight the spread of this last enemy, world fascism. His new perspective altered his opinion of old friends as well as old ideas. Disillusioned and alone Bethune turned his back on his former life. He was "totally disenchanted with . . . urban life. He found it corrupt and infinitely boring . . . . [He] was well along to becoming tough mentally. He was beginning to blot out all of the nonsense and small talk that was so much a part of any cultured person's life in the west at that time and now."

Several days after the Japanese had captured Peiping

in August, 1937, Bethune was speaking in Salmon Arm, British Columbia. After the meeting, he talked with members of the local Spanish Aid Committee and told them he had decided not to return to Madrid. The real struggle was in China, and he would join it there. He seemed bitter. "They call me a Red .... If Christianity is Red, I am ... a Red. They call me a Red because I have saved 500 lives," he said in Timmins. In September, near the end of the tour, he approached Tim Buck to ask for his support. Buck telephoned Earl Browder, the Chairman of the American Communist Party, to determine what arrangements could be made with the Chinese. Buck and Browder were willing to help Bethune but the Communist Parties in both Canada and the United States were heavily committed financially to the war in Spain. Browder consulted William Dodd Jr. of the American League for Peace and Democracy and Philip J. Jaffe, publisher of *Asia Today*, an American left-wing periodical. Jaffe, who had just returned from China, was extremely enthusiastic about helping the Communists and was in the midst of preparing an organization for that purpose called the China Aid Council. The prospects of financial backing for Bethune looked good.

The decision to go to China was the most formative of his career. Canada for him was an empty homeland; Spain had ended in regret. At the age of 47, his personal life had reached a close: Frances had been gone for years; his affairs with other women were fruitless and sad; he had no close friend, apart from Barnwell, whom he seldom saw; he had no child, and his family was part of the past. He was alone.

Frances said he went to China "for a last fling." He saw there a new chance to justify his whole life, serving in a revolution he sensed was one of the most important in history.

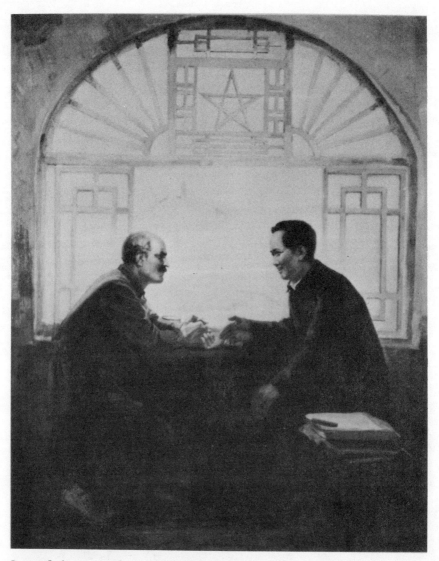

One of the most famous posters in China, this shows Bethune, with
a Leninist look, meeting Mao Tse-tung in Mao's cave at Yenan, April
1, 1938. In the background is the Yenan pagoda, symbol of Communist
Chinese resistance to the Kuomintang and the Japanese.

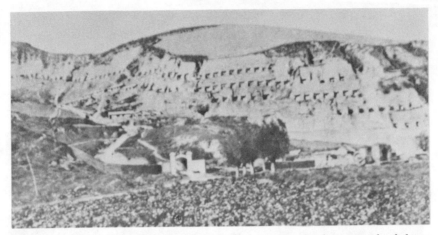

Bethune worked in the cave hospitals in Yenan, photographed here in 1938 or 1939. After his death the Chinese renamed the complex the Norman Bethune International Peace Hospital in his honour. The caves are now used as family homes.

Bethune met General Nieh Jung-chen (centre) with a Chinese journalist in Wu-t'ai in June, 1938.

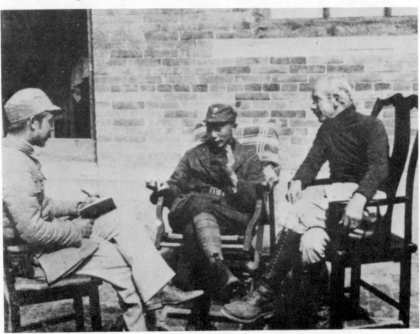

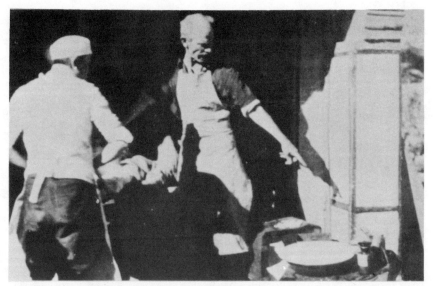

Bethune operates in a Buddhist temple, probably in Hopei in 1939.

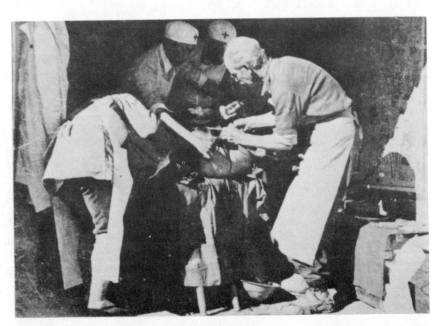

The best known photograph of Bethune in China, taken the same day as the preceding photograph. This was reproduced on a postage stamp issued by the Chinese government in his honour. Bethune, characteristically operating without gloves, is wearing Chinese peasant sandals.

Operating in the field, Bethune bends over a patient carried straight from battle on a wood stretcher.

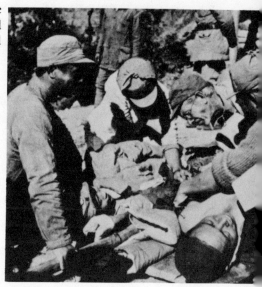

Bethune rode through central China at the head of his medical team on a white horse captured from the Japanese and presented to him by General Nieh.

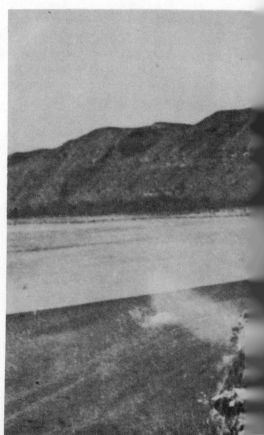

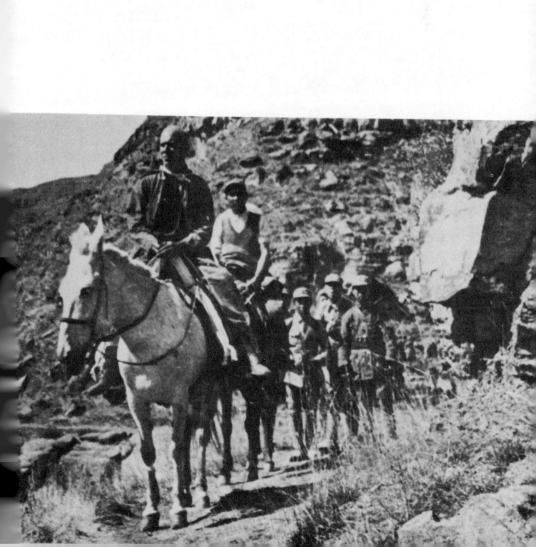

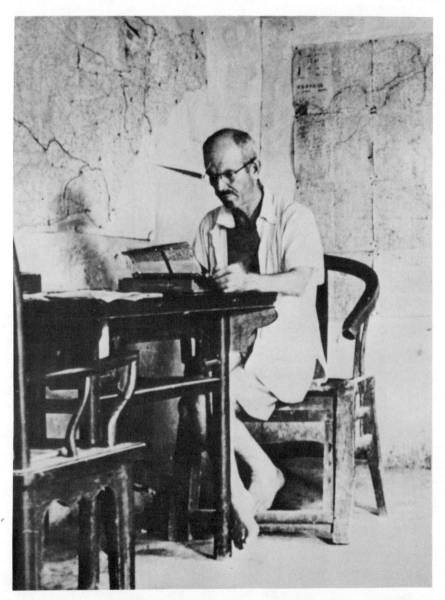

Bethune wrote textbooks, letters, stories and articles while at the front in China. The typewriter was one of his few personal effects, and is now in the Bethune museum in Shih-chia Chuang.

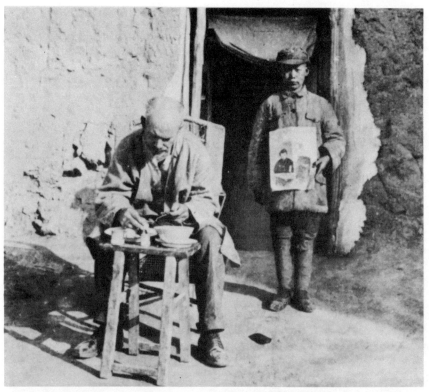

Bethune's *hsiao-kuei* (personal aide), Ho Tzu-hsin. Ho had trouble learning to cook eggs for Bethune, and when he succeeded, Bethune celebrated with this photograph. Ho holds up an English language magazine.

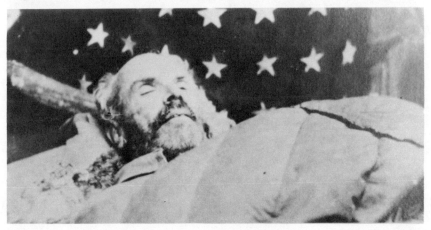

When Bethune died, the Chinese could not find a Canadian Red Ensign or a Union Jack, so they draped his bier with the Stars and Stripes.

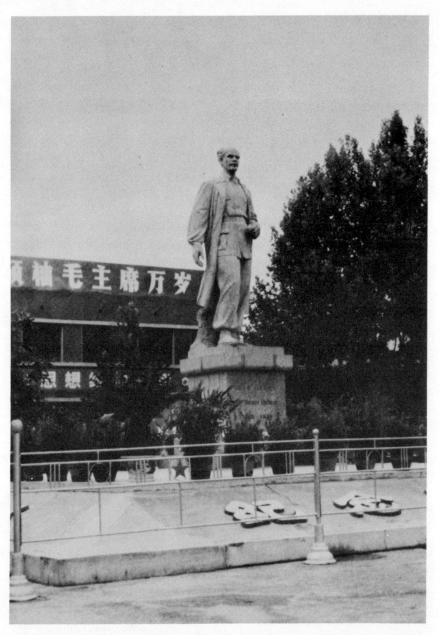

Bethune's statue stands before the Norman Bethune International Peace Hospital in Shih-chia Chuang. Another statue is near his grave in the Park of the Martyrs' Tombs of the Military Region of North China.

Huan-ying, Huan-ying

On July 7, 1937, as Bethune was speaking in Timmins, Ontario, Japanese troops opened fire on Chinese forces in the walled town of Wan-p'ing near Peiping. This Lü-Kou Ch'iao (Marco Polo Bridge) Incident was the opening salvo of the Second Sino-Japanese War.

The first Sino-Japanese War had begun on September 18, 1931, with another "incident" at Mukden in Manchuria. Eager for land and ready for battle, the Japanese invaded Manchuria, drove out the Chinese, and took it over as the puppet state of Manchukuo. General Chiang Kai-shek, leader of the most powerful army in China, virtually ignored the invaders and concentrated all his efforts on the so-called "bandit-suppression" campaign against the small durable force led by Mao Tse-tung. For five years in the south and centre of their country Chinese fought Chinese while the Japanese gradually extended their rule over the north. In 1936 a group of Chinese intellectuals formed the National Salvation League, the forerunner of the United Front. Chiang Kai-shek, faced with rebellious officers, a discontented army and a disastrous military situation on every front, was finally forced to join in the United Front with Mao's Communists. On September 22, 1937,

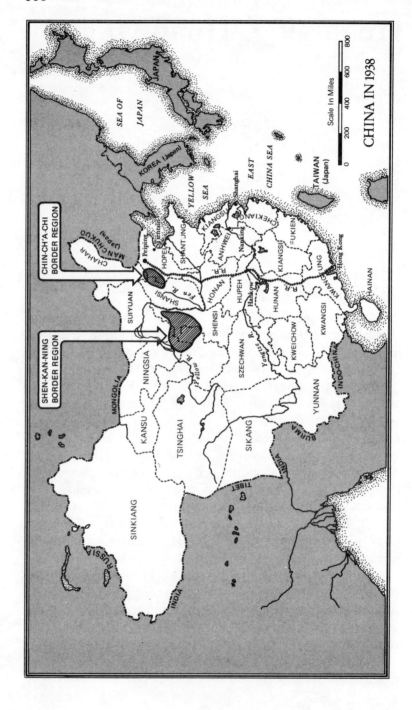

CHINA IN 1938

the Kuomintang-Communist United Front was publicly announced. The Chinese, weak and poor, turned to face the invaders behind a bare facade of unity.

The Japanese held much of the north and the former capital, Peiping. Bethune read the reports in the newspapers and talked about the situation with his friends. They saw China as they had seen Spain, a first line of defence against the growing power of world fascism. In both countries, according to the communist analysis, the classic struggle had begun. The propertied establishment was waging civil war against workers and landless peasants, covering up the class struggle with the mask of nationalist sentiment. In both cases, the capitalist-bourgeois elements profited from foreign intervention to defend their system. Bethune, along with the others, identified the Japanese, Kuomintang, Spanish Falangists, Italian Fascists and German Nazis with decadent imperialist capitalism under the single title, world fascism. In this analysis, there was no significant difference between Spain and China. Mao Tsetung was one great leader among the world fighters against the fascist threat.

Bethune went to New York in October of 1937 where he received a guarantee of some financial support from the C.A.C. and the A.L.F.P.D. Both organizations advised him to seek funds from private sources as well, and he turned for help to New York officials of the Committee to Aid Spanish Democracy. Among them he met a recent medical graduate, Dr. Lewis M. Fraad, who offered to accompany him to China. Fraad, a New Yorker, knew some wealthy liberals interested in China, and set out with Bethune to raise the money. By Christmas they had approximately $5,000, to which was added $1,000 from the China Aid Council. Bethune decided to buy enough equipment to outfit an entire base hospital. As funds were made available they toured various medical supply and drug companies, buying goods and storing them in a New York warehouse.

By Christmas, 1937, the unit had two new members.

Jean Ewen, daughter of a prominent Canadian Communist, was asked by the Canadian Communist Party to join Bethune. A registered nurse, she had practised in a Shantung hospital for two years and spoke Chinese. She was not a Communist, but was young, intelligent and sympathetic to the Chinese cause. She came to New York to meet Bethune, Dodd and Jaffe and agreed to go to China. The other volunteer was Dr. Charles H. Parsons, a capable American surgeon who had worked and taught in the Wilfred T. Grenfell Medical School in Twillingate, Newfoundland. Unfortunately Dr. Parsons was fighting a losing battle with alcohol. Bethune regarded Parsons as a qualified risk but in his evangelistic optimism reasoned that he could probably be converted.

They were all busy with telephone calls, rushed visits to potential donors, haggling for discounts on medical supplies and the preparation of inventory lists. A member of the Spanish Aid Committee who helped Bethune prepare for the trip described him:

> All of us felt he was going to his death. We knew what conditions were there. He was going to cut himself off at his age from modern medicine . . . . There was no fanfare and he wasn't the hero from Spain. He was sitting around the warehouse . . . and the boys were really thinking [it] through with him. What kind of saddle-bags? How much medicine? It was grim. He was very business-like. He never showed anything. I would go home and cry.

The trip to China was far different from that to Spain. There was little interest in Asian affairs because everyone was absorbed by developments in Spain. The committees backing Bethune had raised little money and seemed unable to generate much publicity. Bethune was alone again:

> It did enter all our heads . . . . Would any of us have done it without the compelling reasons that might make anyone a hero? Would anyone have gone to the lengths that he did to go there unless he had already said goodbye to many things here? He was very lonely at the end. The decision

put a kind of space around him. By that time we had quite a few people who believed in Spain, who worked ... got wounded ... and died for Spain. But China was different. It wasn't our culture. It wasn't our anything.

On New Year's Eve, 1937, a farewell party was held for Bethune in New York. The next day he and Parsons left by train for Vancouver, where they met Jean Ewen. Dr. Fraad, who at the last minute could not go with them, explained why: "I never did get to China. Bethune had to leave without me because I was ... denied a passport. Bethune died without ever knowing why I did not meet him in China. My letters probably never got to him. He wrote to me twice asking indignantly why I did not appear .... They were short notes, somewhat angry." In Vancouver the three members of the Canadian-American Mobile Medical Unit boarded the S.S. Empress of Asia on January 8, 1938, for their nineteen-day voyage to Hong Kong. On board ship Bethune wrote several last-minute notes. To Frances he said: "I am doing what I can for you, for justice and my former love for you. I am giving you what is due you. Please do not consider it any other way except that." To Marian Scott he wrote:

> You see why I *must* go to China. Please read *Edgar Snow's* book—Red Star over China ... *Agnes Smedley*—Red Army Marches, *Bertram's* First Act in China.
>
> I feel so happy & gay now. Happier than since I left Spain.
>
> Goodbye & bless you
Beth
Goodbye again, comrade

The doors were shut on the past.

Trouble began among the three soon after they left Vancouver. Perhaps because the money was American, Parsons headed the unit. Jean Ewen describes him:

> He was a peculiar sort of character. Bald-headed, very quiet with a marshmallow face. No distinctive characteristics or

features .... He didn't even try to be reasonable with
Bethune nor was Bethune any better to him .... I think
I felt rather sorry for Parsons—he just didn't have a clue
on how to function as a social human being. As long as
he had a bottle—nothing else mattered.

Because Bethune feared that Parsons was using the unit's
money in the ship's bar, he urged Ewen to join him in
sending a telegram to New York to demand that Parsons
give a financial accounting. She refused until they reached
Shanghai when a telegram was jointly sent to the League
for Peace and Democracy to insist on Parsons' recall.

When their first contact failed to appear in Hong Kong,
Ewen sent a telegram to Agnes Smedley, who urged them
to fly to Hankow. They had just exchanged greetings with
Smedley at the Hankow airport when the air-raid alarm
sounded and everyone rushed for cover. Hankow, the
temporary capital of China after the savage "Rape of Nan-
king" by Japanese forces in December, 1937, was under
constant aerial attack. After the all-clear, they were invited
to stay at a private home called the "Yenan-Heaven Axis."
The large stone house was the residence of Bishop Rootes,
an ultra-liberal American Episcopalian who opened his
doors to all progressives.

Their plans had been vague when they left Vancouver
and their only instructions were to make themselves available to the Chinese government, who would decide where
they would be most effective. The attempt to determine
their ultimate destination brought about the final clash
between Bethune and Parsons. Dr. R.K.S. Lim, Director
of the Chinese Red Cross, made some suggestions but was
interrupted by Bethune who declared emphatically that
he had come to China to serve in the Chinese Communist
Eighth Route Army and would go nowhere else. Parsons
refused to go north with the Communists, so Bethune and
Ewen set out alone. Parsons went back to the United States
with all the remaining money.

Bethune and Ewen met Chou En-lai, later Premier of
China, and Chin Po-ku, Co-ordinator of Medical Supplies
for the Eighth Route Army, on their first day in the Rootes'

home. Both Chinese were stationed in Hankow as Communist representatives during the period of the United Front. Chou and Chin, invited to have coffee with the foreign medical personnel, were delighted to learn of Bethune's determination to serve with the Communist forces. While Chin Po-ku was making the necessary arrangements to guide the two Canadians north, Bethune demanded that he and Ewen be put to work during their enforced stay in Hankow. They were willingly accepted for surgical duties in the Presbyterian mission hospital in the neighbouring city of Han-yang.

Bethune was invited to several dinners in Hankow restaurants attended by missionary doctors and newspaper men. At one of these he met an English journalist, James Bertram, who gave Bethune his sleeping bag, riding boots and fur cap. He described Bethune:

> He was then very tense and strung up—smoking heavily and obviously under considerable strain.... He... wore a small pointed beard à la Lenin, and liked to strike a Lenin pose when being photographed.... I thought him a very lively and gifted man, but pretty egoistic and certainly driven by a daemon of his own; he wanted to be a hero or a martyr of the Revolution, at any cost.

After three weeks, the final preparations had been completed for their journey north to Chin-kang K'u, the headquarters of the Chin-Ch'a-Chi Border Region in mountainous Shansi province. Chin-Ch'a-Chi (Shansi-Chahar-Hopei) and Shen-Kan-Ning (Shensi-Kansu-Ningsia) were the two military areas controlled by Communist forces. Under normal conditions, this trip of more than 800 miles required several days. But Japanese troops were advancing from the north-east towards the strategic Peiping-Hankow rail line on which they set off, and no one knew if they would get through.

The train filled with merchants and students left Hankow on February 22 and arrived in Cheng-chou that night. The city was crowded with refugees fleeing from the advancing Japanese troops, and they were forced to sleep in a railshed beside the station. The next day the train to Tung-kuan was stopped and evacuated several times as Japanese planes flew overhead. In Tung-kuan they waited thirty-six hours in an empty mail car for the train to Lin Fen. Bethune was angry at the increasing number of delays and had been drinking heavily. To pass the time he produced a ukelele from his baggage and began to sing accompanied by their guide, who turned out to be an accomplished harmonica player.

Word had reached Hankow, meanwhile, that Lin Fen was about to fall to the Japanese. The International Red Cross sent out a missionary doctor, Robert McClure, to warn Bethune and Ewen. As McClure was riding his bicycle around Tung-kuan, a revolver strapped to his waist, he found Bethune near the railway station. The meeting was extraordinary to McClure. For two Canadian doctors, both graduates of the University of Toronto, to meet in northern China in the middle of a war would normally have led to some recognition of their common background. Bethune found no cause for celebration, according to McClure:

> He didn't feel himself a Canadian. He felt that he'd given up Canada. He was very critical of the establishment.... They were all money-grubbers, they were status-chasers. Very paranoid about anybody in thoracic surgery, particularly [because] they had ostracized him and had not recognized his ability. They had kept him out of practice, kept him out of the jobs that he wanted to do. They thwarted him in his efforts to establish his brand of thoracic surgery in Canada. Very bitter.

Bethune was far more interested in discussing the future than the past: "He was fighting in the world revolution. The Spanish front had closed off and he was going to the China front."

The meeting with McClure had little effect on Bethune—he did not even record it in his diary. He was determined to go to Lin Fen despite McClure's warnings. On the way they passed several trains heading south packed with refugees. When they arrived, Japanese troops were

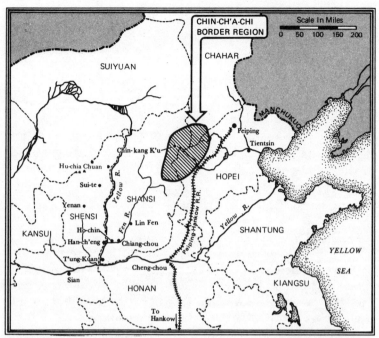

only a few miles from Lin Fen, and a complete evacuation
was taking place. As the town came under heavy aerial
bombardment, trains left for Tung-kuan with people cling-
ing to the roofs of the cars. In the confusion their guide
could not find the local Chinese military unit, and he urged
them to go back to Tung-kuan. Bethune had no choice.
Within minutes they were on a freight train, propped up
on rice sacks, heading back south. A few hours later the
train stopped and they could hear angry voices. Ewen went
down the line of cars to discover that the engineer had
left the train, refusing to continue along the heavily
bombed line. Once more there was confusion. At last it
was decided that mules would be bought from the people
in a nearby village to carry the train's valuable cargo of
400 bags of rice. The two Canadians had no choice. They
joined the mule train of forty-two carts that was headed
in almost the opposite direction to their original destination. In the late afternoon two Japanese bombers spotted
the mule train and descended to a level of 200 feet to
drop their bombs. While everybody ran for shelter, the

mules remained on the road. Bombs killed 18 of them. After the Japanese left, they unhitched the carts from the dead mules, transferred their cargo to those remaining and resumed the march.

Travelling all night they reached the Fen River where they rested for several hours and ate before crossing to the city of Chiang-chou. As they waited for barges, a small line of people began to form outside the peasant hut where Bethune had been sleeping. The word had passed quickly in the village that a foreign doctor had arrived and they spent several hours treating the sick. When they entered Chiang-chou, Bethune wrote:

> I climbed up the hill, through the city, to the church. The city is practically deserted except for fat shopkeepers and beggars. These two classes are all that remain—the propertied and the propertyless. The first will await the coming of the Japanese with some fear and trembling but their goods are more important than their fears. They are the typical bourgeoisie the whole world over. They regard this war as just another battle between professional soldiers. They are politically illiterate. Their only concern is their individual welfare.

At the top of the hill they met two Dutch Franciscan priests. During the conversation they offered Bethune a cigar and opened a bottle of wine. One of the priests later bade them goodbye with the words, "I hope we meet again on earth, if not, then in Heaven."

As they travelled west from Chiang-chou, they learned that the advancing Japanese cavalry were barely twenty-five miles from the city. The Japanese, like the fleeing Chinese, were heading down along the Fen River towards the Yellow River, some thirty miles away. All along the route they met refugees who joined their caravan. Ignoring the protests of others, Bethune was constantly stopping to attend to the sick and the wounded. At one point, a young soldier no more than sixteen years of age caught Bethune's eye as he lay beside the road. His shoulder was smashed to a pulp, and he cried, "I don't want to die, I have not lived." When the quarter-master warned Bethune that he was delaying the mule train, Bethune angrily turned on him to remind him of his duty to the wounded. He hastily did what he could for the boy and rejoined the caravan.

They reached Ho-chin on March 3 to find it filled with the provincial troops of General Yan Shi-san in retreat less than a day ahead of the Japanese. The press of civilians and soldiers recreated the now familiar confusion they had encountered along the way. Forced to remain in Ho-chin overnight, Bethune " . . . walked in the town. Live carp in water buckets for sale, black pigs with big floppy ears; barkless dogs; white paper windows! . . . My birthday—48—last year [I was] in Madrid. Dressed six wounded soldiers (arms and hands) nothing but neglected minor injuries—all others have died on the way back." They arrived at the Yellow River the following evening:

> Here was an unforgettable sight. Lit by a dozen fires five thousand men were collected with trucks, carts, mules, horses, artillery and great piles of stores waiting to cross the river into [the province of] Shensi. The light of the fires was reflected back from the steep wall-like mountain side. The river rushes between two high cliffs.
>
> The swift current (12 miles an hour) carries great floating ice floes which clash against each other far out on the dark surface. The whole scene is wild and fantastic.

They crossed the river the next day as the Chinese dug trenches and built emplacements for light artillery and machine guns. In the late afternoon the Japanese arrived on the east bank while Chinese fugitives were still crossing the icy waters. They opened fire on two junks in mid-stream laden with women and children, and their screams could be heard by the Chinese who angrily returned the fire from the opposite bank. That night Bethune and Ewen took refuge in a cave. In the morning, with snow falling, the Japanese artillery arrived and shelled the Chinese for three days. Unable to move because of the bombardment, they were forced to wait for the Eighth Route Army trucks to drive them to Sian. Bethune attended to the civilians in the cave:

> Woke to hear one of our Chinese singing the Marseillaise. A fine clear day with sharp wind. A child with convulsions—terrified mother, soap-stick enema cure! During the convulsions the mother rushed outside the cave and called the child's name loudly. This to bring back his soul which had temporarily left the body (reminds me of the Scotch "bless you" when one sneezes).

During their enforced confinement, Bethune and Ewen spent the evenings around a campfire and he talked of his life before China. Ewen recorded her opinions of him:

> We had come a long and tortuous road together. I felt I knew him well, but I was in for many surprises before we parted .... It was here I met the Doctor's wife, Frances, the light of his life .... How wonderful he thought her.
> He was in himself very unhappy; in his personal life he could not make the adjustments required of adults. He did not accept himself or his limitations; irascibleness touched with arrogance made him unapproachable ....
> In his work with the sick and the wounded, I saw only a man dedicated to the service of all mankind .... Compassion for suffering humanity he had in abundance, and would go out of his way to help a patient as I have not seen many doctors do ....
> He lacked understanding of the other fellow's point of view. He felt he was right, or rather that Marx was right .... He firmly believed that the Marxist doctrine alone imbued men with compassion and a sense of duty.

When the trucks did not arrive, they set out on foot and reached the city of Han-ch'eng on the following day, March 10. Here they were assured that trucks were expected at any moment from Sian. Their request for work was gratefully accepted. They operated in a military base hospital and treated a steady stream of civilian patients until March 19 when the trucks finally arrived to take them to the ancient walled city of Sian. When they arrived on March 22, they went directly to the Headquarters of the

Eighth Route Army. Under the agreement of the United Front the Communists had been permitted to maintain an administrative unit in Sian. Until Chiang Kai-shek began to break the spirit and the principles of the United Front, the Sian headquarters remained a vital part of the Eighth Route Army apparatus since it served as a national recruiting centre. From all parts of China, young men and women made their way to Sian. Here they were interviewed and learned the nature of the hardships they would have to face in a guerilla war. Those prepared to endure then received passes and continued north to the central base of all Communist forces at Yenan.

After hearty handshaking and many smiles, the Chinese ironically congratulated them on returning from the land of the dead. Apparently the North American newspapers in Hankow had reported them missing and believed killed after the Japanese had taken Lin Fen.* Of far more consequence to the two tired travellers than their reported deaths was the welcome offer of a bath. After that, a second delight awaited them. In an old Buick brought out of storage in their honour they were driven to the Sian Guest House where they were the dinner guests of two Swiss doctors. An excellent European-style dinner was served on a linen tablecloth with silver service, and they lingered over coffee and brandy talking to their hosts, Dr. Hermann Mooser and Dr. Heinrich von Jettmar, members of the League of Nations Epidemiological Unit stationed in Sian. Back in Eighth Route Army Headquarters they were introduced to Chu Teh, Commander-in-Chief of the Eighth Route Army. Jean Ewen described the meeting between Chu and Bethune:

[Chu] had a powerful handshake. He was well into his fifties,

*Canadian and American newspapers reported this on March 12, 1938. Four days later, March 16, they were reported to be in Sian. Bethune states that they arrived in Sian March 22. According to him they were in Han-ch'eng from March 10 until March 19. It is possible that Eighth Route Army officials in Han-ch'eng informed Hankow of their arrival and their destination of Sian. Since Bethune maintained a methodical and accurate account it seems unlikely that his chronology was in error, especially by six days.

his kind face wrinkled and weather-beaten. His generous mouth spread in a broad grin of welcome as he embraced Dr. Bethune. Both at once said "Let me have a look at you," each in his own language—Chinese and English. Then Chu walked round and round Dr. Bethune, both laughing heartily, admiring each other as only men do when they feel they both measure up.

For the next few days Bethune and Ewen held meetings with the League of Nations Unit to arrange for the transfer of medicines and supplies which Dr. Mooser agreed to turn over to Bethune. These formed a valuable addition to their own supplies which had been stored in a Hong Kong warehouse since January. Their concern for them ended when Dr. Richard Brown, a Canadian Anglican missionary, arrived in Sian just before they left for Yenan. Brown, driven out of his mission in Honan by the Japanese, had gone to Hankow to establish a refugee centre. There he had learned of Bethune and Ewen and had been persuaded by Bishop Rootes to join them. Brown brought welcome news that the medical supplies had been taken from Hong Kong and were en route to Sian under Eighth Route Army guard. Of equal importance to Bethune was that Brown, an experienced surgeon who spoke Chinese fluently, had agreed to join the unit. Bethune was overjoyed. On their last day in Sian, Dr. Chiang Chi-tsien, Director of Medical Services for the Eighth Route Army, arrived to accompany them north.

Before dawn on the morning of March 28, a fleet of trucks began the journey to Yenan, more than 200 miles north of Sian. The first fifty miles led over a dirt road bordered by fertile fields. Gradually the farmland disappeared as they entered the dry brown loess hills, and they could see clearly the numerous natural terraces and caves formed by years of erosion. The trip took three days. At nightfall they entered the dusty town lying in the shadows of the surrounding hills beside the Yen River. High above the town was the Yenan pagoda, which became the symbol of this island of resistance against both the invading Japanese and later the Kuomintang. It was here that the exhausted Communist forces led by Mao Tse-tung and Chu Teh set up headquarters at the end of the Long March in 1935. After the United Front agreement with Chiang Kai-shek in September, 1937, Yenan had become the military, medical and administrative centre of the Eighth Route Army, part of the National Revolutionary Army.

As the trucks pulled to a halt, a man approached on a bicycle, stopped and extended a hand of welcome. He spoke English. Known as Ma Hai-te to the Chinese, he was George Hatem, an American who had arrived in Yenan in the summer of 1936 where he had remained as one of the very few trained physicians in the Eighth Route Army. While rooms were being arranged for Bethune and Ewen in the Yenan Guest House, Dr. Ma took the pair for a dinner of noodles at a cooperative restaurant followed by coffee, captured from the Japanese, in Ma's cave.

Toward midnight a messenger appeared at the Guest House to announce that Mao Tse-tung wished to see them. Bethune dressed quickly and they followed the messenger. Inside the Communist leader's cave, lit by a single candle, they saw a tall man dressed in the blue cotton uniform of an ordinary soldier. Seated at the table was his secretary and interpreter. "The tall stern figure came toward us smiling and in a rather high-pitched voice . . . greeted us with 'Huan-ying, huan-ying,' (welcome, welcome). He held out both his hands to Dr. Bethune who accepted his greeting in a like manner." During the discussion that continued into the early morning hours, Bethune gained a clear picture of the military-medical organization that supplemented what he had learned earlier from Dr. Chiang. Mao, meanwhile, was eager to learn of Bethune's experiences in Spain in order to determine to what extent he could duplicate his effort in China. Bethune explained that Dr. Mooser and Dr. Yang Yung-mien of the Chinese Sanitary Corps in Sian had promised money and supplies for the establishment of a hospital in Yenan to complement the existing Border Region Hospital managed by the Eighth

Route Army. Mao strongly objected to this plan, pointing out that, despite the inadequacies of the Yenan hospital, the need of additional medical assistance was greater at the front in Shansi. They finally decided that until a working arrangement could be hammered out among the Communists, the League of Nations Unit stationed in Yenan and the Sanitary Corps, Bethune would be most useful working in the Border Region Hospital.*

His jubilation at meeting Mao lasted for days, and Bethune began planning for his work at the Border Region Hospital. Everyone in Yenan was aware that a foreign doctor was in their midst, the first to come since the Japanese invasion. During the next several days he attended banquets in his honour and was invited to speak to the students of K'ang-ta, the Yenan military academy and university. Bethune told them about the Spanish war and attempted to describe the various shades of Canadian and American opinion concerning the aggression of Japan, Germany and Italy.

Bethune and Ewen were moved from the Yenan Guest House to the caves which extended as far as thirty feet into the sides of the loess hills. Along one side of each cave was a *k'ang,* an upraised clay or brick stove-bed topped with straw, beneath which a fire could be lit. The dry caves with their rounded ceilings were relatively warm in the winter and cool in the summer. Bethune's equipment was moved to a cave and he was assigned his *hsiao-kuei* (little devil), a combination guard, valet and messenger. Ho Tzu-hsin, a seventeen year old standing only a shade over five feet in height and weighing under one hundred pounds, was chosen. When Ho first saw Bethune he was frightened and ran away, but an interpreter brought him back

*The Sanitary Corps, financed by and responsible to the Kuomintang Government, was attached to the League Unit. When Yenan appealed to Hankow for medical aid, the latter placed certain conditions on this aid which would force some of it to be used for civilians in Yenan. The Communists felt that their priorities were for medical aid to their troops in the Chin-Ch'a-Chi Border Region. Bethune, unaware of the details, was simply informing Mao of the apparent desire of the League and the Sanitary Corps in Sian to build a second Yenan hospital.

and introduced him to Bethune. Ho remembers the first meeting: " . . . I came into his cave. There were two caves. Bethune's possessions were placed in an inner cave. How was I to arrange them? Bethune took my hand and showed me where to place various things and helped me carry the iron cot which was too heavy for me. Then he showed me several times how to arrange his cot before he left." A *hsiao-kuei* was also expected to cook, but Ho had little experience: "Every morning I prepared his breakfast and he taught me how to boil an egg. When once I pleased him by boiling the egg exactly as he liked it he gave me a book and I stood beside him. We had our picture taken with him eating the egg from a bench and me holding the book."

Since the Yenan leadership was still unable to reach an agreement with the League Unit and the Chinese Sanitary Corps, Bethune began to work in the Border Region Hospital. The conditions appalled him. The hospital consisted of approximately fifty caves cut into the hillside. The patients slept without sheets, huddled together in their soiled and tattered uniforms on the dirty matted straw that covered the two or three *k'ang* in each cave. Electricity was available only in the operating room and sanitation measures were almost non-existent. The caves were connected by an outside path and during the rainy season the steady flow of water down the hillside made passage from one cave to another virtually impossible.

After a few days under these conditions, Bethune protested loudly. He demanded changes the hospital officials were unable to carry out. Angered and sulking, he returned to his cave and refused to work until his demands were met. Although he had participated in two wars, he had never seen anything like this. He was completely unprepared for the primitive conditions that existed in Yenan and those he later found at the front:

He'd sit down and discuss things and argue things and he'd get awfully impatient. Then he'd have to cool down a little and we'd start all over again . . . . The realities of the Chinese situation, the political, the material, the medical situation were entirely different than any concepts that he had . . . . So for us who were here on the spot, he was thinking in terms . . . [that] didn't fit and when you'd argue with him, his impatience would get the upper hand.

Finally Bethune's concern for the sick and wounded quelled his impatience and he returned to work.

When it became clear to him that no agreement on the projected hospital would be reached, he saw his chance to be closer to the Shansi front where he felt he could be more useful and satisfy his desire for action. His original idea of repeating his Spanish experience had been negated by Chinese conditions. Lack of electricity for refrigeration, the poor condition of the roads and the distance to the front made him realize the futility of such a plan. More viable and hence more appealing to the Yenan leadership was his suggestion to form a mobile medical unit to operate near the front. Here his Spanish experience was relevant and he argued persuasively that he could save many lives by going to the wounded rather than waiting for them to make the long journey to Yenan for medical attention.

Eventually Mao and Dr. Chiang agreed to send a unit consisting of Bethune, Ewen and Brown to the Chin-Ch'a-Chi Border Region. On May Day, 1938, the truck loaded with medical supplies and food stood outside the hospital. The Canadians were moving.

I Have Found
My Mission in Life

Bethune went out to the truck that was to take the unit north. Seated in the back beside the ten wooden crates of supplies was their escort of twelve fully-armed soldiers. When he failed to find Ho Tzu-hsin among them he reacted swiftly. "Where is Ho? He must come with me," he told the startled officers. A little afraid of this demanding foreigner, they began to discuss what to do. While they talked, Bethune went to find Ho himself. Ho recalls the incident: "To guard him the Party appointed some strong soldiers. Bethune told the Party that he did not need them. Instead, he wanted only me, his *hsiao-kuei*. He then came to the cave and took me to the truck, picking up my knapsack. From that day I remained with him until his death."

Two months after they had first set out from Hankow, they took the road heading north and then east to Chinkang K'u, the mountain headquarters of the Chin-Ch'a-Chi Border Region. The route leading through the barren loess hills was enhanced by a narrow tributary of the Yellow River which ran along beside the road. Rain greased the clay surface and forced them to reduce their speed. Near Sui-te, the road became a quagmire and trapped the truck. After fruitless efforts by the driver to move, Bethune jumped from the cab and looked at the rear wheels mired in the mud. With the pouring rain soaking his yellow windbreaker he signalled the driver to move forward. Then, to the astonishment of the Chinese, he stepped ankle deep into the mud and began to push. One of the soldiers was incredulous: "It was so unlike a foreigner to get dirty." The following day they reached Sui-te where they spent the night. Here Bethune wrote a letter which contradicted the impression he had given McClure: "We call it the Canadian-American Medical Unit, but that's just to let the Americans get their money's worth—all three of us are Canadians!" At the end of the road mules were rounded up and the precious medical supplies were transferred to wooden boxes designed to fit their backs. Bethune and Brown passed the day treating nearly thirty wounded soldiers.

All along a rugged narrow mountain trail cut by eight rivers Bethune and Brown treated civilian patients in isolated villages. At night they slept in peasant homes, and Bethune would set up his cot on top of the clay *k'ang*. Their food was supplied by the peasants: millet or rice, vegetables, a little meat, eggs, all washed down by gallons of tea. Bethune frequently had Ho prepare his favourite speciality, steamed potatoes mixed with eggs and covered with sugar. He had left Yenan in civilian clothes—a tie, a pair of slacks, yellow sneakers and his yellow windbreaker. In one village he found several uniforms of the Eighth Route Army and asked permission to be fitted with one. Strutting proudly between two mirrors Ho had placed on opposite walls, he glowed: "Look at me, almost fifty, and I'm a soldier once more."

After more than five days of tiresome walking over craggy treeless terrain, they reached the tiny village of Hu-chia Chuan 20 miles west of the Yellow River, the site of an Eighth Route Army base hospital Dr. Chiang had asked Bethune to inspect. Without resting they conducted a thorough examination of the patients, staff and facilities. Bethune was shocked and infuriated by what he saw. The pitiful condition of the wounded, the untrained staff and the appalling lack of supplies and medicine were beyond his imagining. The full import of the Chinese situation began to penetrate his mind but instead of sulking as he had in Yenan he immediately set to work. For three days the two Canadian doctors prepared an operating room and a post-operative ward. From their own supply of cotton cloth they made sheets, towels, gauze squares, masks and glove cases. The hospital held 175 wounded, of whom 35 were serious:

> All have old neglected wounds of the thigh and leg—most of them incurable except by amputation. Three of the 35 are lying naked on straw-covered k'angs with only a single cotton quilt. The others are still in their old, unwashed, cotton-padded winter... uniforms. They are, without exception, all anemic, underfed and dehydrated.... They are dying of sepsis. These are the cases we are asked to operate on. They are all bad surgical risks.

Despite the risks, Bethune and Brown operated for five consecutive days on the fifteen most seriously wounded. Only one patient died.

During those first days at Hu-chia Chuan, Bethune was busily planning the reorganization of the medical facilities. In what he described as a "brief introductory report on medical conditions... with some recommendations for your consideration," he presented a detailed critique of existing conditions. There were four glaring weaknesses in the base hospital. Primary among these was the lack of sanitation: "Food is left exposed to flies; dressings, after removal, are thrown on the floor, instead of into a receptacle; the patients are not washed; cross infection is the rule not the exception. Two of our cases developed maggots in their wounds within 5 days after operation." The second problem was the obvious inability of front-line medical personnel to treat the wounded properly. Improper care of many of the Hu-chia Chuan wounded had significantly reduced their chances of recovery even before they had reached the rear hospital. The third problem concerned the medical training of the hospital staff. Bethune was unwilling to operate on many patients simply because none of the nurses understood the techniques of post-operative care. Finally he pointed out not only the deficiency in facilities and medicine but the incorrect choices of medicines on hand, many of which were not needed. All these weaknesses he believed could be eliminated with the adoption of three basic recommendations. The first involved training of the medical staff. The second was the construction of a supply route from Hankow to Yenan and thence to Hu-chia Chuan to bring in the required medicines. The third was the establishment of a hospital closer to the front.

Bethune still had not fully understood the reality of the situation. He suggested that nurses and doctors be sent to Hankow and other cities not under direct Japanese attack to be trained by Mission Hospitals and the Chinese Red Cross. Under existing wartime conditions the arrangement of their transportation alone would be a serious problem. Nor did he sense the fragility of the United Front. Arguments between the Communists and the Kuomintang had resulted in Chiang Kai-shek's refusal to allow Red Cross supplies to be sent to Yenan. Even if a supply route around the Japanese lines could be devised, there were no funds to provide "the tenfold increase of all medical supplies" demanded by Bethune. Lack of money also prevented the construction of special hospitals near the front.

It took some time for Bethune to adjust to the military and political facts of the war. On this adjustment hinged his usefulness to the Chinese cause. Although he was unable to recognize at first the full complexity of the problems, he did understand that his plans could not easily be translated into action. He therefore outlined a limited short-range course of action in his report. He and Brown would leave Hu-chia Chuan for an inspection tour of the front. There they would be able to determine the general condition of the Eighth Route Army Medical Service and give front-line instruction on the treatment of wounds. At the end of the tour, Brown would have to go since his leave was almost over. Bethune encouraged him to arrange another leave from his Anglican mission and proposed in the meantime to form a mobile operating unit. He ended his report from Hu-chia Chuan with a lament that would be echoed throughout his letters and reports during the next eighteen months. He had heard nothing from his American backers:

> I have exhausted every means in my power to try and get a word from the American Committee. I give it up—after 5 months... we have no money to cable... and even though we had, our experience in the past has been so disappointing that I don't feel like asking the Eighth Army to give us the money to try again.... I have sent the American Committee enough material for publicity and press to fill a paper. The only reply was a letter from the mail clerk of the American League for Peace and Democracy asking me if Yenan was my correct address. But not a line from anyone else.

Here was another obstacle that left some of his carefully devised schemes stillborn in his notes. Parsons left with the initial funds, and the further financial support he had been promised from America never arrived.

They remained sixteen days in Hu-chia Chuan. On May 27 the unit struck out eastward, stopping along the way to treat the sick and wounded. In the late afternoon of June 17 they arrived at Chin-kang K'u in the heart of the Wu-t'ai area of north-eastern Shansi and within sight of the Great Wall of China on the border with Hopei. They were met by Nieh Jung-chen, the thirty-nine year old Commander-in-Chief of all Communist forces in the region. Bethune was in good spirits:

> The first thing he did was raise his fist to the brim of his cap in a strange salute. We asked him if this was the Canadian salute, but he replied, "No, it's a combination of the Spanish and Chinese salutes: in Spain they raise their fist, and here you put your palm to your cap-brim; I've combined the two." Everyone laughed at this.

After the warm greetings, Nieh suggested that Bethune go to the quarters assigned to him and rest before supper.

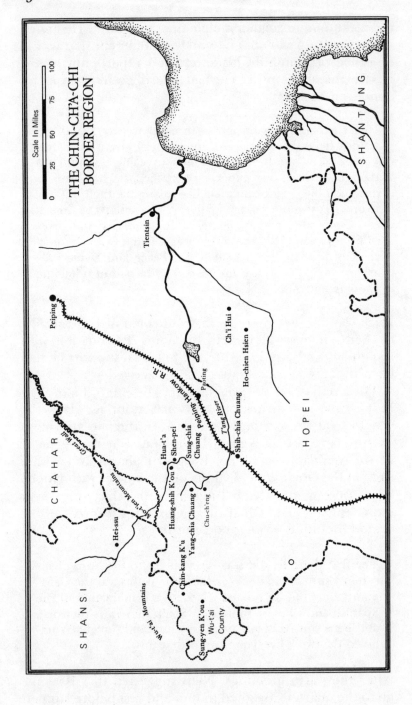

THE CHIN-CH'A-CHI
BORDER REGION

Scale In Miles
0   25   50   75   100

SHANTUNG

Tientsin

Peiping

Ch'i Hui

Ho-chien Hsien

HOPEI

Paoting

Hankow R.R.

T'ung River

Shih-chia Chuang

Sung-chia Chuang
Peiping

Hua-t'a
Shen-pei

Great Wall

Mo-t'ien Mountains

CHAHAR

Huang-shih K'ou

Yang-chia Chuang
Chu-ch'eng

Hei-ssu

Chin-kang K'u

Sung-yen K'ou
Wu-t'ai
County

Wu-t'ai Mountains

SHANSI

Suddenly Bethune's mood changed. Speaking sharply, he stated that he had come to work, not to rest and eat, and brusquely demanded to be taken immediately to the hospital. An embarrassing few moments followed as Nieh explained that the wounded were a full day's ride from Chinkang K'u. Finally Bethune was persuaded to eat and spend the night. Early the next morning the unit set out for the nearest hospital. They arrived at 5 p.m. and once more the Chinese urged him to rest and eat before examining the wounded. Bethune was adamant as he had been the day before. At 11 p.m. he returned from an inspection tour of the facilities and patients, then sat down to dinner.

Conditions at the three hospitals in the Wu-t'ai area were much the same as at Hu-chia Chuan but Bethune was better prepared this time. He spent the first week examining patients, preparing case histories and classifying them into treatment categories. For the next twenty-five days he and Brown operated on 110 cases. When they were not operating, the two Canadian doctors gave daily classes to the medical staff, organized "clean up squads," instituted a fly-control plan and even found time to direct construction of a recreation park for the walking wounded. "Things are going well," he wrote to Ma in Yenan, "a combination of shouts, tears and smiles has worked wonders here."

Brown left in the middle of July, planning to return in late October. Bethune was alone and faced with an awesome responsibility.* To an American friend he wrote: "We are completely surrounded by the Japs, north, east, west and south. They hold all the towns on the railways, but we still retain the enclosed country. In this great area of 13,000,000 people and with 15,000 armed troops, I am the only qualified doctor." Instead of being intimidated

*Jean Ewen had returned to Sian for supplies for the Yenan Central Hospital before Bethune and Brown left for Wu-t'ai. Upon her return to Yenan she worked as the Head Nurse in the hospital there. Bethune wrote to her advising her not to follow them because of the adverse conditions. She later worked in Lan Hsien, then returned to Canada before Pearl Harbour and never saw Bethune again.

by his circumstances, he was enthusiastic and optimistic. In the same letter he requested his friend to ask Dr. Fraad to come to China, remarking that "We—that is, the 3 of us—Brown, Fraad and myself, can have a wonderful time here."

Given the conditions in which he was forced to work, only an idealist could survive. Peasant homes served as wards. There were no sheets, no electricity, no sanitary precautions, few medicines and fewer instruments. Bethune himself had more instruments than the entire medical service of the Eighth Route Army, and he had exhausted the supply of medicines he had brought to China. He set up headquarters at Sung-yen K'ou and put into immediate action a plan he formed during his first few days there. His first step was to create conditions in which he could work with existing facilities. In addition to designing and supervising construction of an operating room, he designed and helped build a sterilizer, leg and arm splints and dressing trays. Under his direction an incinerator and stretcher racks were constructed and a de-lousing sterilizer was planned.

Before his arrival there had been only haphazard organization of the staff. He created a routine, beginning with a conference every Sunday afternoon of the combined medical and nursing staff at which responsibilities could be assigned and problems discussed. The duties of the nursing staff were defined, printed and posted on the walls. Before each conference every patient was visited in ward rounds and his progress noted on his report. Because patients were in various peasant homes, each was given a metal disc with his name and number. A master list and a map showing the location of all patients were kept in Bethune's office.

Both in Yenan and Hu-chia Chuan he had noted the low level of training among the medical personnel. In Wu-t'ai it was the same. There were no graduates of medical or nursing schools and very few had received any formal training. Since most were intelligent, dedicated and eager to learn, Bethune decided to teach them himself. With the aid of his interpreter Tung Yüeh-ch'ien, he held lectures every other day from five to six in the afternoon. He began with the fundamentals of medicine, teaching basic anatomy and physiology. Always aware of the practical objectives of his instruction, he taught them how to treat simple wounds. In July he started to write a medical text to supplement his lectures. All these developments, outlined in his report of July 20, had taken place in less than a month. They were part of his "Five Weeks Campaign" to produce "the finest hospital in the Eighth Route Army."

The immediate results were pleasing to Bethune, the staff and the patients. In one vital respect, Bethune's spirit was congruous with that of the Eighth Route Army. Poorly equipped, badly clothed and underfed, they were united by a fanatical desire to drive out the invading Japanese. Well prepared by their ten-year war against Chiang Kai-shek's army for the struggle against Japan, the Communists, like Bethune, were pragmatic in their approach. They ignored tradition and custom, and this freshness of mind made them receptive to Bethune's improvisational genius.

Bethune recognized the similarity. For the first time in his life he felt he was working together with people in a united effort. He amazed the Chinese by showing as much concern for the welfare of the peasants as he did for the soldiers of the Eighth Route Army. When he visited a village where many persons were suffering from a skin disease, he ordered construction of large wooden vats to hold fresh water. Then he and his assistants bathed the diseased and applied an ointment he had improvised. Within three weeks most of the afflicted were cured of an ailment that had plagued them for years. In another village, seeing a young girl with a harelip, he stopped and explained to the child's mother that he could eliminate her daughter's impediment. He found a suitable peasant home and immediately performed the operation. Relations were not always so smooth. Bethune's old inner enemy impatience frequently dominated him, to the perplexity of the Chinese. Nurses and orderlies would approach Brown and say

"What's wrong with Dr. Bethune today? He's so cross. He's throwing his instruments around."

Until Bethune arrived most Chinese had never witnessed a blood transfusion and were extremely reluctant even to be typed. Bethune would demonstrate the painlessness of blood extraction by removing a small amount of blood from his assistant or himself. On one occasion, needing blood quickly, he ordered some of his assistants to hold an unwilling donor from whom he extracted the required amount:

> As soon as he got the right antigen, he didn't explain to the poor fellow. He said, "He'll do. Bring him along." So they grabbed him and made him lie down. He started to struggle a bit, so two or three held him down. Bethune got his little apparatus into one vein, and another end of it into the vein of the receiver and the blood transfusion was complete. It was a bit forceful, but it was complete. I might say it didn't help the rest to volunteer, the way he was treated.

Bethune had reduced his demands for supplies so that the Chinese could meet them. When he was told that the constant threat of Japanese troops made it impossible to guarantee regular delivery of supplies, he exploded in fury. General Nieh recalled:

> When Dr. Bethune came to the area he and we did not at first understand each other. He went around criticizing this and that. He felt that we were working in an unenlightened way. We felt that he did not appreciate the difficulties under which we laboured. There was a gap between us.

One of these gaps grew from Bethune's desire to begin a medical school. During the Five Weeks Campaign he approached Nieh with the proposal for a "model hospital" at Sung-yen K'ou, in addition to the base hospital already there, to be used as a training area for doctors and nurses in the Wu-t'ai area. The initial reaction of Nieh and the army leadership was negative. Bethune wanted the hospital to be permanent, and they feared it would be vulnerable to Japanese attack. Bethune persisted, pointing out the desperate need for trained personnel. Finally, rather than offend him, the Chinese agreed.

In the village was an unused Buddhist temple set in a grove of willow and pine trees on a rocky hill above the road. Under Bethune's direction, three hundred peasant families from the village carried stone and lumber to the site and built a thirty-six bed hospital. Carpenters made the wooden beds. Peasant women made straw mattresses, cloth sheets and blankets. Bethune himself joined in the labour, which lasted nearly two months. During the construction period Bethune prepared a curriculum for the medical training school. In a telegram to the Yenan Military Council on August 11, he announced that the school would open in a week. To maintain its operation he requested a monthly sum of $10,000 and a further sum of $5,000 which was needed immediately for medicines. He also stated that a pamphlet outlining the treatment of wounds would be published shortly. Meanwhile he was working on a larger book with more than 200 drawings to be used as a basic medical text for the training school. He expected to complete the text in three weeks.

Two days later he changed his plans. General Nieh had urged him to accept the principalship of the school but Bethune strongly resisted, pointing out that part of his time should be spent at the front improving treatment of the wounded. He told Nieh: "The best way ... is to go to these doctors and instruct them in the field under actual conditions." Instead of the three-week deadline predicted two days earlier, he estimated that he needed two more months to complete his textbook. During this time he would continue to instruct the staff using the Model Hospital at Sung-yen K'ou. When the book was ready for publication in mid-October, he would combine his proposed inspection tour and front-line instruction.

Bethune's arguments convinced Nieh. Although it was true that Bethune sometimes lost his temper and had still not completely understood the nature of a guerilla war, Nieh knew that all his schemes were designed to help the wounded. It was also difficult to be critical of a Westerner who insisted on being fed the same food as the Chinese soldiers and who was angry on learning that he had been assigned to better living quarters than they. Nieh recognized that this was indeed a unique foreigner. When he informed Bethune that the Yenan Military Council had authorized an additional monthly salary of $100 for him, Bethune telegrammed the Military Council:

I refuse to accept offered $100 a month .... Have no need of money personally, as all food, clothing, etc. is supplied me. If this money has been sent to me personally from America or Canada, make a Special Tobacco Fund out of it for tobacco and cigarettes for the wounded. I will draw from time to time what little money I need from Headquarters here.

Even if there had been somewhere to spend the money he would not have had time for his former pleasures. His textbook alone took several hours every day. When he was not writing, operating or instructing, he worked with the carpenters and stone masons on the temple-hospital at Sung-yen K'ou. He summarized his feelings in a diary entry of August 21, 1938:

I have operated all day and am tired. Ten cases, 5 of them very serious .... It is true I am tired but I don't think I have been so happy for a long time. I am content. I am doing what I want to do .... Why shouldn't I be happy—see what my riches consist of. First I have important work that fully occupies every minute of my time from 5:30 in the morning to 9 at night. I am needed. More than that—to satisfy my bourgeois vanity ... I have a cook, a personal servant, my own house, a fine Japanese horse and saddle. I have no money nor the need of it—everything is given me. No wish, no desire is left unfulfilled. I am treated like a kingly comrade, with every kindness, every courtesy imaginable. I have the inestimable fortune to be among, and to work among, comrades to whom communism is a way of life, not merely a way of talking or a way of conscious thinking. Their communism is simple and profound, reflex as a knee jerk, unconscious as the movements of their lungs, automatic as the beating of their hearts. Here are found those comrades whom one recognizes as belonging to the [upper] hierarchy of Communism—the Bolshevists. Quiet, steadfast; wise, patient; with an unshakable optimism; gentle and cruel; sweet and bitter; unselfish, determined; implacable in their hate; world-embracing in their love.

The Model Hospital was opened with great ceremony September 15, 1938, but Bethune spent very few days in it. When the Japanese launched an offensive in Hopei province, he hastily put together a mobile unit and rushed to the front. He was on horseback throughout October, riding through the mountain region of West Hopei instructing and operating. During this trip he learned of the complete destruction of the Model Hospital by Japanese troops who attacked Sung-yen K'ou soon after he left, less than three weeks after the hospital's inauguration. It was a bitter blow to Bethune, but it also proved correct the Military Council who had feared this very possibility. The costly lesson helped him understand the nature of the war, and he returned to his original plan of developing mobile units.

The Japanese September campaign had already forced him to form one mobile unit consisting of Bethune, two Chinese doctors, Tung, his interpreter, whom he had trained as an anaesthetist, an operating-room nurse, a cook, two orderlies, and two *hsiao-kuei*. Their equipment included a collapsible operating table designed by Bethune, surgical instruments, antiseptics, twenty-five wooden leg and arm splints, ten iron leg and arm splints, sterile gauze and medicines. All this was carried on three mules. As the fighting continued and the winter snow began to fall, Bethune's unit remained in West Hopei, riding from battle to battle. There was little time for rest. On November 20 he arrived at a base hospital and, after examining the wounded, operated until midnight. With only four hours of sleep he led his team across mountain trails so deep in snow they had to dismount and walk beside their horses. They ate and slept in peasant villages along the way. At one of these he found two gangrenous soldiers who had worn tourniquets for three days. Had there been medical attendants at the battle this could have been avoided. Bethune severely criticized the army commander, Wang Chen, and made him promise to warn him in advance of their next planned action so that Bethune's team could be stationed directly behind the troops to give immediate help.

Bethune finished the inspection tour and returned to Yang-chia Chuang, his new headquarters. In late November Wang Chen advised him of a planned attack against the Japanese and asked him to ride to Hei-ssu, a mountain village close to the front. Bethune arrived and set up an operating room in a small temple surrounded by cypress trees. Their only protection against the sub-zero temperature was a sheet for a roof and a blazing fire near the operating table. They were eight miles from the nearest attacking regiment and fifteen from the farthest. Aided by a well-organized stretcher unit the wounded began to arrive, and for the next forty hours, Bethune and his two assistants, Dr. Yu and Dr. Wang, operated on 71 soldiers. On the evening of November 30, two doctors arrived to give Bethune, Yu and Wang some rest. After only a few hours sleep, they returned and continued to operate until ten the next morning. Two days later he was at a base hospital almost thirty-five miles away inspecting the wounded who had been taken there from the battle.

The inspection of the wounded and the organization and performance of his unit at Hei-ssu exhilarated him. Because he had been able to set up the unit in position before the battle, the first patient was received only seven hours after having been wounded. The longest time was forty hours and the average twenty-four. In the past, most patients had received no attention for days. He was also delighted by the low infection rate. In spite of having been carried nearly thirty-five miles, twenty-two patients escaped infection entirely. The most significant result was that one-third of the soldiers were able to return to action within a month. In terms of guerilla warfare this was an outstanding achievement.

After several months of struggle, Bethune had at last begun to develop an efficient portable system suitable for Mao's army. He made this very clear in his monthly report to General Nieh:

> We have demonstrated to our own satisfaction and I hope to the satisfaction of the Army commanders the value of this type of treatment of wounds. It is expected that it will revolutionize our present concepts of the duties of the Sanitary Service. The time is past and gone in which doctors will wait for patients to come to them. Doctors must go to the wounded and the earlier the better.

The Hei-ssu experience convinced Bethune that with mobile operating units forming the basis of the Sanitary Service, thousands of lives might be saved. Units could be stationed at base hospitals from which they would follow their regiments into action—to be effective each regiment would need its own mobile unit. To carry out this plan he would have to establish a new training school and complete his medical text. On December 7 he returned to Yang-chia Chuang to work on these projects.

Although he had been in China for less than a year, he was already a legend. The name of Pai-ch'iu-en was known to every soldier in the Chin-Ch'a-Chi Border Region.* Stories of his selflessness and extreme dedication to the sick and wounded had spread among the troops. They told of how he had given away his clothes to the wounded at Hu-chia Chuan and how he had once ridden 17 miles to look after one soldier at the front and returned immediately to his base hospital.

During the fall of 1938 he was appointed Medical Advisor to the Chin-Ch'a-Chi Border Region. He was, in effect,

---

*It has been suggested that the Chinese transliteration of Bethune's name means "White Seek Grace" or "White One Sent". These meanings can indeed be given to the Chinese characters, but this is entirely coincidental.

in command of all Chinese Communist medical forces, working night and day, rushing to battles, operating, returning to sketch plans for the mobile service, snatching moments to write a few pages in his medical text or a letter to Canada. He sometimes woke from a dead sleep, left his cot and began to type. His new interpreter, Lang Lin, awakened by the noise, asked why he couldn't wait until morning. Bethune replied, "Something's on my mind now. It will be gone by morning." The members of his medical team vainly begged him to slow down and explained their fears for his health to an Eighth Route Army Commander. When the officer politely and formally suggested to Bethune that he rest, Bethune angrily replied that he was responsible only to General Nieh. Word did eventually reach Nieh, who spoke to Bethune. When Bethune rejected his advice, Nieh ordered him into a room to sleep for six hours. Bethune grumpily lay down on a *k'ang,* then suddenly jumped up, snatched a cigarette from Nieh's lips and hurled it to the dirt floor. Glaring at Nieh he shouted, "In respect to medical matters, I will not take orders, even from you," and stomped out of the general's headquarters. Minutes later he was in the operating room.

His responsibilities weighed heavily on him. He believed that he was the representative of progressive elements in Canada and perhaps all North America and that his work in China would symbolize the internationalist spirit of communism. In a speech at the opening of the Model Hospital he said:

The eyes of millions of freedom-loving Canadians, Americans and Englishmen are turned to the East and are fixed with admiration on China in her glorious struggle against Japanese Imperialism. This hospital has been equipped by your foreign comrades. I have the honour to have been sent as their representative. Do not consider it strange that people like yourself, thirty thousand li away, half way around the globe, are helping you. You and we are internationalists; we recognize no race, no colour, no language, no national boundaries to separate and divide us.

This had a powerful impact on the isolated Chinese, fighting for their lives and country against a powerful invader. His presence inspired them to believe that others equally concerned would soon come to their aid. Bethune felt drawn much closer to the Chinese than he had ever been to the Spaniards. In the same speech he remarked: "I used to think of it as 'your' hospital, now I think of it as 'our' hospital. For between us we have created it."

The spirit of comradeship with the Chinese was important and helpful in his work, but Bethune still could not speak the language, he was without friends and China was not home. He felt the loneliness of his exile. Only a few friends in North America wrote letters to him and those took months to arrive:

I have not seen an English language newspaper for over 6 months with the exception of the Japan Advertiser of April 15 left behind by the Japanese in a Shansi village. I have no radio. My isolation is complete. If I did not have enough work to fill 18 hours a day, I would certainly feel discontented.

Will you do this for me? Just one thing! Send me 3 books a month, some newspapers and magazines. I won't ask you to write letters. I would like to know a few facts—"Is Roosevelt still President of the United States? Who is Prime Minister of England? Is the Communist Party in power in France?" Some other facts would be welcome also—"What is the China Aid Council doing for China, for the 8th Route Army? How much money have they sent? Are they sending more doctors or technicians? Am I to have assistance? Am I to have the medical supplies I have been asking for 5 months?" I have exactly 27 tubes of catgut left and ½ lb. of carbolic acid. I have one knife and 6 artery forceps—all the rest I have distributed. There remains 2 ½ lbs. of chloroform. After that is finished we will operate without anaesthetics. Now for Marx' sake, get busy!

... All the above would seem that I was complaining bitterly of my lot. On the contrary. I'm having a swell time.

With Comradely greetings
Norman

A few weeks later in a homesick letter to friends in Canada, he described the conditions under which he was living:

> My life is pretty rough and sometimes tough as well. It reminds me of my early days up in the Northern bush. The village is like all other Chinese villages, made of mud and stone, one-storey houses, in groups (families) of compounds. Three or four houses are enclosed in a compound facing each other. In the compound are the pigs, dogs, donkeys, etc. Everything is filthy—the people, their houses, etc. I have one house to myself. It has a brick oven running along the single room. In this I have my cot and table. I have made myself a tin stove in which is burnt coal and wood. The windows (one) are papered with white paper. The floor is packed mud, so are the walls . . . . Let me confess that on the 1st of the New Year I had an attack of homesickness! Memories of New York, Montreal and Toronto! If I were not so busy I could find reasons enough for a holiday.
> With the kindest remembrances of you all . . . .

He was far too busy to complain strenuously. In December he turned to the question of building a mobile medical service. His plans were to bring one Sanitary Service representative from each of the subdivisions of the Chin-Ch'a-Chi Border Region to Yang-chia Chuang to take an intensive three-week course. He would teach the duties of a doctor, nurse and nurse's assistant working under battle conditions. These selected representatives would then return to their sub-regions to instruct the other Sanitary Service personnel. On January 3, 1939, thirty representatives from the various sub-regions attended the Special Surgical Practice School. It was hardly the type of training he had expected to introduce in the days of the Model Hospital but it was the best that could be done under the circumstances.

Shortly after his arrival in the Wu-t'ai area he had intended to visit and inspect every base hospital in the Border Region. The Japanese September offensive and the work on the training school had delayed his plans. In February he was at last free to complete his inspection tour and test a larger unit in the field. For the next four months his team was constantly on the move inspecting, setting up brief training courses, and operating under enemy fire. Wherever he went Bethune followed his routine. If he was visiting a hospital for the first time, he made a thorough inspection tour, questioned the director in detail, then called a conference of the whole staff to discuss its method of operation. Here criticisms were made openly by both Bethune and staff members. Following the free discussion, agreed changes became part of the staff's routine organization. He described the personnel of a typical hospital in his diary:

> The doctors who run this hospital range in age from 19 to 22, and not one of them has received any training in a modern hospital; the nurses are young people between 14 and 19. These are our greatest resource: they study diligently, strive to improve themselves, and are willing to listen to criticism. Sometimes I'm unhappy with them from the point of view of medical knowledge, but when I see their purity, their sincere efforts to study, their love of their comrades and their selfless diligence, I can always find a way to suppress my dissatisfactions . . .

The eighteen-member team, which included Dr. Yu Sheng-hua, Deputy Chief of the Chin-Ch'a-Chi Sanitary Service, left Yang-chia Chuang February 19, crossed the Japanese-held Peiping-Hankow railway, and headed for Ho-chien Hsien, the Rear Hospital of Central Hopei. Bethune was mounted on a white stallion captured from the Japanese, a present from General Nieh. Because this was a plains area, they were forced to travel at night in peasant garb to avoid detection. On one occasion they were nearly attacked by a Japanese cavalry troop who galloped after them. The Japanese were gaining when by chance the unit met an Eighth Route Army Regiment which drove off their pursuers and allowed them to reach Ho-chien Hsien. During his inspection of the Rear Hospital, he found the nurses on ward duty wearing face masks and immediately ordered them removed. The head nurse, An Chih-lan, and several other nurses were angered by his demand and complained against the order. Bethune listened carefully as they explained why they wore masks: the rooms were small, the air was often fetid and some of the wounded were diseased. When they had finished Bethune replied: "The wounded have come from the front where they were prepared to sacrifice themselves. Why do you treat them as if they were dirty?... Contagion is not our worst enemy." The nurses removed their masks.

He astonished both nurses and doctors by preparing and cleaning his instruments and the operating room before and after the operation himself, rather than leaving these tasks to the nurses. His singleminded devotion to the patients, especially at the expense of his own health, amazed the Chinese. He would often take his soup into the wards and say in his broken Chinese, "Comrade, how do you feel after the operation?" When the soldier opened his mouth to speak Bethune spooned in some soup. The patients soon learned that he was using his own rations to feed them and they resolved to refuse his offer of food. When Bethune came back the next night, again carrying soup and a spoon, he was greeted by protesting shouts. Lost without his interpreter, he vainly tried to convince a patient to take some soup. The noise attracted several doctors and nurses to the ward. The clamour died down and a doctor explained that the wounded believed Bethune needed his food as badly as they.

On one occasion Bethune was preparing a patient for an operation. He decided that a blood transfusion was needed, and, since none was available, prepared to give his own blood. Ignoring the protests of the nurses and his assistant he lay down on a door that served as a stretcher and ordered them to begin the transfusion. When he had given his blood, he rose and performed the operation. Word spread quickly that the foreign doctor had given his blood for a Chinese. Bethune took advantage of their wonder and proposed that each of the villagers have his blood typed. The type was recorded in a master list of all the villagers. To avoid any error, the type was also recorded on a piece of cloth sewn into the lining of each donor's clothing.

Bethune frequently offered and gave his own blood to patients, despite vigorous attempts by his assistants to prevent him. Once, while an assistant distracted him by arguing that another donor should be found, a nurse and a doctor silently moved a lightly wounded patient into position and completed the transfusion. Bethune was amused and played his own trick on the Chinese. During the lunch hour he would often be operating. When a *hsiao-kuei* arrived with his dinner, Bethune told him to return in fifteen minutes. The boy returned punctually to find Bethune still at work. This continued every fifteen minutes for two hours. Finally, with the nurses laughing openly at the exasperated expression on the *hsiao-kuei*'s face, Bethune accepted the food and was forgiven for his prank. He had never before shown a lively sense of humour, but the trust that had grown between himself and the Chinese allowed him to play comic roles for the first time in his life. He took great pleasure in asking his patients if they would get better. Eager to acknowledge his skills, they replied *"how"*, the Chinese expression for "yes", and never failed to draw a laugh from Bethune.

From Ho-chien Hsien they continued on the inspection tour to Ch'i Hui, where a fierce encounter with the Japanese began on April 26. Bethune set up his operating room in a temple two miles from the front and prepared to receive the wounded. The battle was intense: Japanese soldiers nearly encircled a Chinese battalion before reinforcements arrived and drove the Japanese back. Casualties were high and began to arrive soon after the outbreak of gunfire. At one point Japanese light artillery bombarded the immediate area of the hospital. A shell hit the temple, demolishing part of a wall thirty feet from the operating table. After many hours of steady work, an assistant pleaded with Bethune to rest. He dunked his head in a bucket of cold water for a few seconds and returned to work. The doctors and nurses all urged him to rest, and he did, finally, but for no more than ten-minute intervals. When the Japanese were driven off, the unit had operated for sixty-nine consecutive hours on a total of 115 cases. Long before Bethune made his official report to General Nieh, the story of his endurance at Ch'i Hui had spread across the plains of Hopei and through the mountains of Shansi. Soldiers adopted slogans such as, "We fight at the front. If we are wounded, we have Pai-ch'iu-en to treat us. Attack."

It was undoubtedly Bethune's greatest performance under fire. The fighting in Hopei was savage and whenever the mobile unit was in action it was never more than three miles from the front. But the pace had begun to tell on Bethune. Trudging along snow-covered mountain trails, racing on horseback to battles, eating only millet, eggs, and potatoes and sleeping no more than six hours a night had made him gaunt. He was forty-nine and looked sixty-five. In four months he had performed 315 operations, established thirteen operating rooms and dressing stations, given two training courses and set up two new mobile medical units. In his report of July 1, Bethune said he wanted to form seven more mobile units before the end of the year and later to enlarge them as the nuclei of divisional field hospitals.

Bethune constantly reminded his students wherever he went that a doctor had to possess the skills of four craftsmen—blacksmith, carpenter, tailor and barber. This impressed the Chinese who had watched him work with blacksmiths making iron splints and with carpenters fashioning his collapsible operating table. He also made his own saddle-bags and showed the Chinese how to shave a patient before an operation. During the fighting in Hopei he had found time to develop a carrying device for use by the mounted mobile teams. Many of the medicines in the leather saddle-bags had been destroyed by the rough travel over the mountains, so Bethune designed a wooden case to carry medicine and operating equipment. The device, which contained material sufficient for 100 operations, 500 dressings, and 500 prescriptions, fitted on the back of a

mule and could be set up in thirty minutes. Bethune called
it a *lü-kou ch'iao* (Marco Polo bridge).

He had solved problems of transportation but he could
do nothing about supply. He was once forced to perform
fifteen operations without anaesthetics:

> The supply of drugs is pretty poor in most places in Central
> Hopei. Difficulty is being found in getting supplies from
> Tientsin. The missionaries are being closely watched. One
> lot of drugs was examined on the way by the Japanese
> and when told that they were going to a mission hospital,
> they made a note of all bottles and packages and later
> checked up on the mission. The mission reported that the
> drugs had been "stolen" by the partisans . . . to account for
> their non-arrival.

The Japanese warned all Christian missionaries against
aiding the Communist forces. When the inspection tour
was returning to headquarters, they were attacked by the
Japanese in Sung-chia Chuang. Bethune became so frustrated by the lack of supplies that he resolved to assume
a disguise and go to Peiping to buy medicine. Kathleen
Hall, a nurse who was director of the Anglican mission
in Sung-chia Chuang, was to go with him. His assistants
at first thought he was joking when he explained his plans
to them. When he began to pack his bags, they were horrified and tried to explain that the Japanese would execute
him if he were caught. On the day of his intended departure
he received a telegram from General Nieh ordering him
to report at once. Nieh made it clear to Bethune that under
no circumstances would he be allowed to risk a trip to
Peiping, no matter how badly supplies were needed. All
Bethune's arguments were in vain, and Kathleen Hall later
told Dr. Ma that he returned "like a shame-faced boy"
to confess that Nieh would not permit the trip. Fortunately
she agreed to make several dangerous journeys to Peiping
herself before the Japanese discovered her activities and
burned her mission to the ground. Her contribution was
of paramount importance to the Sanitary Service. At various times she brought a total of $15,000 worth of drugs

to Bethune, enough, he predicted, to supply the Chin-
Ch'a-Chi Border Region through the winter of 1939–
1940.*

The tour continued its return home and stopped in
Shen-pei, where Bethune wrote the July report in which
he said " . . . the education of the doctors and nurses of
this region is the main task of any foreign unit." By mid-July
he had completed a draft outline of the medical school
with a planned initial class of 100 students. The course
for nurses would last six months, for doctors eighteen
months and for surgeons two years. He also proposed the
creation of a model hospital to be used to train the students.
To establish this he requested a sum of $2,000 plus oper-
ating expenses of $3,000 monthly. During the remainder
of July he continued preparations for the medical school
and completed his third book, *Organization and Technique
for Divisional Mobile Operating Units,* with 150 pages and
50 illustrations.

At Shen-pei Bethune reflected on his work during
the past year. As outstanding as his own personal contribution had been he realized that he would be unable
to continue operating as a front-line surgeon, inventor,
writer of medical texts and teacher. His greatest value
would lie in the development of his proposed medical
training school. Foreign units were desperately needed
in China and their worth would be measured by the
skills they could teach the Chinese. The failure of his
American sponsors to supply him with the needed funds
deeply disappointed him:*

*Miss Hall continued performing humanitarian work until her death
in the late 1960's. She spent her last years working among the Maori
people. The Chinese government honoured her contribution to their
cause by inviting her on a tour of China in 1966.

*No files could be located of either the China Aid Council or the Ameri-
can League for Peace and Democracy to determine whether any contributions were ever sent to support Bethune. Philip J. Jaffe, the founder
of the China Aid Council, wrote to the author: "Wm. Dodd Jr. of
the American League Against War and Fascism [sic! It was changed
to 'For Peace and Democracy' in 1937. R.J.S.] was assigned to follow
through with help and advice, but Bill was remiss in his duties and

The China Aid Council seems to its China representative in the field to be rather neglectful. I have received 3 letters from them in 20 months. The last was received on January 14th, 1939—over 7 months ago. That letter was mailed from New York on Sept. 20th, 1938. As a result, I am completely in the dark as to the American developments, money, supplies, etc. It is really on account of this ignorance that I am forced to come back. Why have they kept me so uninformed? Perhaps it was too much to expect that some of the individual members of the Council should write me but why had not the secretary done so officially? That I think is not unreasonable.

By August, 1939, he had decided to return to Canada and raise the necessary funds on a speaking tour:

I am leaving this region to return to America about the first week in November if I can clean up my work.... I must make a fast inspection trip of all hospitals (20 now) before leaving.... I plan to be away in America for 3 or 4 months, returning next summer. I must have a guaranteed $1000 [in] gold monthly for this region alone. I'm not getting it. I don't know where the money from America is going to. I can get no information from... America, so I'm going to find out for myself.

He was tired. In August he tried to minimize his declining physical condition: "My health is pretty fair—teeth need attention, one ear has been completely deaf for 3 months, glasses for eyes need correction, but apart from these minor things and being pretty thin, I'm OK." In September he developed an abscess on his thumb which he showed to Lang Lin. When Lang insisted on calling one of the assistant doctors, Bethune curtly refused. Reaching over to his

Dr. B. was fully justified in his complaints from Yenan." Wm. Dodd Jr. is no longer alive. It has been suggested that the Kuomintang intercepted mail for Yenan. Actually the United Front continued to function into 1939 and Bethune mentions a letter that arrived from the China Aid Council in that year. Certainly the Council and the League received mail from Bethune, who sent numerous letters and cables to them. Other letters were received as late as 1939 by North Americans from Bethune. Jaffe's statement would, therefore, seem sound. Bethune was let down.

instrument case, he grasped a scalpel, handed it to his apprehensive interpreter and said, "It's easy. One, two, three." Lang hesitated until Bethune looked sternly at him and he lanced the abscess. Bethune recovered but the experience should have warned him.

Bethune was also lonely during these months. He wrote to his old friend, John Barnwell:

> It's a fast life. I miss tremendously a comrade to whom I can talk. You know how fond I am of talking. I don't mind the conventional hardships—heat and bitter cold, dirt, lice, unvaried familiar food, walking in the mountains, no stoves, beds or baths. I find I can get along and operate as well in a dirty Buddhist temple with a 20 foot high statue of the impassive-faced gilded God staring over my shoulder, as in a modern operating room with running water, nice green glazed walls, electric lamps and a thousand other accessories. To dress the wounded, we have to climb up on the mud ovens—the k'angs. They have no mattresses, no sheets. They lie in their old stained uniforms, with their knapsacks as pillows and one padded cotton blanket over them. They are grand. They certainly can take it. We have had tremendous floods this summer. It's been hellish hot and muggy. Rain for 2 months coming down like a steady shower bath turned on full.
>
> I am planning to return to Canada .... I want to raise a guaranteed $1000 (gold) a month for my work here. I am not getting it. They need me here. This is my region. I must come back.
>
> I dream of coffee, of rare roast beef, of apple pie and ice cream. Mirages of heavenly food. Books—are books still being written? Is music still being played? Do you dance, drink beer, look at pictures? What do clean white sheets in a soft bed feel like? Do women still love to be loved?

Bethune administered to himself the most effective antidote for his loneliness—work. He prepared his mobile team for a final inspection tour of the twenty base hospitals, and supervised the final arrangements for the opening of the medical school and model hospital in Niu-yen K'ou. He was present for the ceremonies on September 18, 1939.

a year and three days from the opening of the hospital at Sung-yen K'ou.

Bethune cut short his inspection tour in mid-October and returned to the front, leading his team along the icy tracks to the foot of the Mo-t'ien mountains where the regimental commander had prepared a peasant home as an operating room. Here he unpacked his instruments and supplies from the *lü-kou ch'iao* and waited for the wounded. On October 28 the team had been operating for several hours when a soldier with a broken leg was brought to Bethune. During the operation his hand slipped and the chisel he was using sliced into the middle finger of his left hand. It was not an uncommon accident. He stopped, allowed a nurse to bandage the wound, and continued to operate. Several days later he was operating on a soldier whose head injury had not been treated for days. Bethune slipped his bare fingers into the deep wound. He seldom wore rubber gloves even when they were available, explaining to his assistants that gloves reduced the sensitivity of the fingers needed in many operations.

Three days later he began to feel tired and weak. He was accustomed to battle fatigue, work exhaustion and travel weariness, but this was something unusual. On November 5, his finger was swollen and he was feverish. The following day an abscess appeared in his armpit. He heard guns in the distance and ordered an assistant to prepare his horse. Waving aside several nurses who pleaded with him to stay, he left the hut accompanied by a furiously protesting assistant and rode through the snow to the front. Five days later he wrote to Lang Lin:

On the north bank of Tang Ho near Hua Ta, West Hopei, November 11, 1939.

I came back from the front yesterday. There was no good in my being there. I couldn't get out of bed or operate. I left Shih Chia Chuang (I think) Hospital of Central Hopei troops on 7th. Pan and I went north. I then had infected finger .... Reached Tu Ping Ti late at night .... We go over west and joined at 3rd Regiment sanitary service on 8th about 10 li east of Yin Fang. Had uncontrolled chills and fever all day. Temp. around 39.6 C., bad. Gave instructions I was to be informed of any abdominal cases of fractured femur or skull cases . . . . Next day (9th), more vomiting all day, high fever. Next day (10th) regiment commander (3rd Regiment) instructed I be sent back, useless for work. Vomiting on stretcher all the day. High fever, over 40 C. I think I have either septicaemia from the gangrenous fever or typhus fever. Can't get to sleep, mentally very bright. Phenacitin and aspirin, woven's powder, antipyrin, caffeine, all useless.

Dr. Ch'en arrived here today. If my stomach settled down will return to Hua Pai Hospital tomorrow. Very rough road over mountain pass.

I feel freely today. Pain over heart—water 120–130.* Will see you tomorrow, I expect.

Norman Bethune

Bethune contracted septicaemia from the soldier with the head wound who had dermatocellulitis, a highly dangerous streptococcus infection.

Members of the team took him to the village of Huang-shih K'ou in the hope that a last desperate operation could be performed. Bethune refused. He knew that he was going to die. During the early hours of the morning of November 12 he slept fitfully, waking to ask for news of his mobile team and to give orders to the doctors and nurses who stood helplessly in a tearful vigil waiting for the end. Shortly after 5 a.m. he coughed and moved his lips in a vain effort to speak. His breathing became weaker. At 5:20 a.m. he was silent.

He died as he lived, lonely and in combat.

*It is impossible to explain this clearly. The figures 120-130 probably refer to his pulse rate.

The Legend

They carried him for four days along the icy mountain paths to a small village where his body remained in a temporary grave until early January, when they moved it to Chu-ch'eng. Near the bier they placed some of his instruments and a few personal effects. Wreaths sent from many miles away surrounded him and above and behind his head were linked the Chinese and American flags, the latter because they could not find a Union Jack. On January 5, 1940, 10,000 persons silently shuffled by the frail gaunt corpse weeping and clenching their fists. He was buried on the side of a hill. By the grave they erected a mat shed in which they hung the wreaths and inscriptions of tribute. On the wall they placed his photograph and in the centre on a pedestal a circle of burning candles to represent the completeness and light of his life. In the evening they staged a play to illustrate his service to the people of China.

The following day the villagers of Chu-ch'eng began to build his tomb. There were no masons and they lacked cement so they walked thirty miles to a quarry to bring back marble at night through the Japanese lines. On May 1, 1940, their work completed, they held the dedication ceremony. A statue of Bethune stood before a globe repre-

senting his international spirit. On each of the four sides
of the base was a quotation about Bethune followed by
the author's name. On the east side was written: "The
Internationalist Spirit of Comrade Norman Bethune is
worthy to be learned and respected by all Chinese people"—The Central Committee of the Chinese Communist
Party. On the south: "The Scientist and Revolutionary of
the Masses"—Nieh Jung-chen. On the west: "The Eternal
Brilliancy"—Tung Yüeh-chien. On the north: "The Most
Valorous Fighter on the Front of the Emancipation of
Mankind"—Lu Tseng-tsao. Several months later, as the
Japanese advanced into the area, peasants removed the
body and the statue and hid them in the surrounding hills
until the Japanese had left. During their brief stay the
enemy troops used the globe for machine-gun practice,
then dynamited it. The Chinese rebuilt the entire memorial.

In 1952, the grave and the tomb were transferred to
Shih-chia Chuang. Bethune remains there in a memorial
park, the site of the Martyrs' Tombs of the Military Region
of North China. The park honours the memory of 25,000
Chinese who fell in the struggle against the Japanese and
the Kuomintang. Bethune's tomb and statue occupy the
prominent position, and a huge pavilion in his honour
is still under construction. Across the road from the park
is the 800 bed Norman Bethune International Peace Hospital. When the tomb was dedicated on May Day, 1940, the
medical school and hospital that Bethune began at Niu-
yen K'ou was renamed the Chin-Ch'a-Chi Border Region
Norman Bethune Hospital. In 1952, the hospital was
moved to Shih-chia Chuang. Its present vice-director is
Chang Yeh-shang, a student of Bethune's at the original
hospital. On the grounds is a museum whose walls display
photographs and line drawings of Bethune's life. In the
centre is a glass case containing his typewriter, several
instruments and some personal effects. Among these are
case histories of some of Bethune's patients while he was
at the Royal Victoria Hospital. Each year hundreds of thousands of people from around the world visit the park and
the museum to pay their respects.

The veneration of Bethune is not hard to understand.

His arrival in Yenan in March, 1938, when the future not only of Mao's forces but of all China was in jeopardy, gave substance to Mao's promise that international Communism would support the Chinese. Bethune was symbolic of the aid to come, but he was more than a symbol. He was a driving organizer whose persistent demand for positive achievement irritated, heartened and inspired the Chinese. During his nineteen months among them, Bethune taught them skills and gave them hope. He performed near miracles by taking peasant boys and young workers and making doctors out of them. He won the admiration of the Chinese by accepting their customs, sleeping in their homes and suffering hardships equally with them. Magnificent as his battlefield achievements were, they were less significant than his personal example of sacrifice and his teaching. At the end, he was working with them almost as equals, and he won their enduring allegiance. To the Chinese, his sole fault was his initial inability to accept the inevitable limitations time and space placed on his far-reaching plans:

His problem of impatience sprang from a sense of not being sure. He didn't know whether he was on the right road or not and he was always searching.... He was committing himself and when he committed himself he was an all-or-none reactor. Only later in the China experience... did he become confident and lose his impatience. At the end everybody began to notice his way of handling the patients, discussing projects, working out plans. There was a certain calmness of spirit that gradually descended upon him.

They understood him from the beginning. If the person's heart was right, then there were no other elements that entered into this. And his aim was always very clear. He wanted to do something for the sick, for the wounded, for the ill, for the dying. And he proved it time and time and time again.... Regardless of what kind of temperament he has, a man who does all of these things... permanently and regularly [makes] the kind of commitment which is political.... Other things can then be handled, be given their proper weight.

General Nieh, who knew Bethune's temper well, commented: "Yes, he was impatient and may have offended some. But during our war this may have had some value. China was then backward . . . . He was impatient with some who were slow and inefficient."

On December 21, 1939, Mao Tse-tung learned of Bethune's death and wrote his famous essay, *In Memory of Norman Bethune*. After the Communist victory over the Kuomintang in 1949, all of China gradually learned about Bethune through Mao's essay. Study of his life became part of the elementary school curriculum. Statuettes and posters depicted him as a heroic figure. Postage stamps bearing his image were issued. During the Great Proletarian Cultural Revolution of the late 1960's, Bethune rose to even greater eminence. *In Memory of Norman Bethune* became one of the "three most read articles" that all Chinese were urged to study and which millions have committed to memory. In an effort to revive the revolutionary spirit among the Chinese people, the Communist leadership chose Bethune as the symbol of selflessness, dedication, and responsibility, characteristics that they wanted to inculcate in the collective Chinese consciousness.

Today in the People's Republic of China Bethune holds a unique position, rare for foreigners in a traditionally xenophobic civilization. Among the more than 800 million people of China only the name of Mao Tse-tung is more familiar than that of Pai-ch'iu-en.

In Canada Bethune's name remained virtually unknown for a generation after he died. Canadians first learned of his death from a terse telegram sent by Chu Teh to the China Aid Council on November 26, 1939, which read: "Unfortunate injury while operating and resultant septicaemia caused the death of Dr. Norman Bethune in Wu-t'ai Shan, China. Eighth Route Army mourns medical hero, and conveys deepest condolences to family and friends." Most major Canadian and American newspapers carried articles briefly outlining his career. Of the few that decided to comment on his amazing life, most concentrated on his political connection with Communism. Except for eulogies in the Communist press and brief obituaries in medical journals, his passing was noticed by few of his countrymen.

There were people who resented this. A handful of friends, medical colleagues and militant left-wingers remembered him and some attempted to gain posthumous honour for his name. In December, 1942, the *Canadian Tribune,* a Toronto Communist newspaper, climaxed a fund-raising campaign with the donation of a mobile blood transfusion unit to the Ontario Division of the Canadian Red Cross. The vehicle, equipped for use in the collection of blood in rural areas, bore the inscription, "Gift of the Canadian Tribune in memory of the late Dr. Norman Bethune." Less than a year later, delegates to the annual convention of the Canadian Congress of Labour adopted a motion to " . . . recommend to the Government of Canada that it take the necessary steps to institute a 'living monument' dedicated to the work of Dr. Bethune . . ." MacKenzie King's Liberal government ignored the recommendation. The first biography of Bethune was published almost a decade later. *The Scalpel, The Sword,* translated into many foreign languages, brought the story of Bethune's life to more readers abroad than in his native country.

For the very few people in Canada fascinated by Bethune, the twenty-fifth anniversary of his death seemed appropriate to tell his story. The Canadian Broadcasting Corporation presented a radio documentary in September, 1964. This was followed by an excellent film biography, *Bethune,* produced by the National Film Board of Canada. For most Canadians the dramatic Bethune of the radio program and the film was appealing, but severe criticism was directed against the federal government for publicizing a Communist. In response to a request of the American Government the Canadian Government stopped distribution of the film to N.F.B. offices in the United States during the late 1960's. Several key persons in the production of the film, enraged by this and an apparent attempt to restrict distribution of the film anywhere outside Canada, considered making it a public issue.

In 1960, the touring Peking Opera Company surprised

officials at Montreal's Royal Victoria Hospital by offering a benefit performance in memory of Bethune. At its conclusion Dr. Ronald Christie, the Physician-in-Chief, suggested to the Chinese that a Sino-Canadian medical exchange would represent a fitting tribute to Bethune. Subsequent negotiations, which included visits to China by Christie, Dr. Lloyd Stevenson, Dean of Medicine at McGill, and the famous neurosurgeon Dr. Wilder Penfield, led to the establishment of the Norman Bethune Exchange Professorship, an arrangement between McGill University of Montreal and the Chinese Medical College of Peking. In 1964, Dr. K.A.C. Elliott, Head of McGill's Department of Biochemistry, went to Peking as the first visiting professor.

Within the next few years, Canadian visitors to China began to report on Bethune's reputation in that country. Most were surprised at being greeted as "countrymen of Dr. Bethune" because they had never heard of him. As late as 1971 the National Historic Sites and Monuments Board, a federally-appointed body with the responsibility of selecting Canadians "of national historic significance", reviewed the qualifications of Norman Bethune and decided that he did not meet the standards. But after Canada and China established diplomatic relations in 1971, there was a sudden change: the Government of Canada decided that the time had come. Recognition of China demanded recognition of Bethune.

At a brief ceremony inside the frame house in Gravenhurst where he was born, Norman Bethune was formally designated a Canadian "of national historic significance." Jean-Luc Pépin, then Minister of Trade, Industry and Commerce, made the announcement before a small group that included Pai Hsiang-kuo, his ministerial counterpart from the People's Republic of China. A similar act was simultaneously being performed in Peking at a Canadian trade fair by the Minister of External Affairs, Mitchell Sharp. The official declaration on August 17, 1972, a generation after Bethune's death, immediately sparked public controversy. For several weeks a heated debate was waged among editorial writers, columnists and the public.

For some, this belated tribute had been unpardonably delayed. For others, recognition of a Communist represented a shocking repudiation of traditional Canadian values. For still others the question was not the fact of paying tribute to Bethune, but the motive. Did the Canadian government truly regard Bethune as a great historic figure or were there more devious reasons? A political cartoon seemed to summarize public opinion: Mitchell Sharp is depicted passing through a Chinese gate carrying a load in a wheelbarrow marked "long-term wheat deal." Outside the wall, an Australian businessman remarks to an American, "The password sounds like Bethune."

Apart from the widely held opinion that the Canadian government had cynically used Bethune to improve commercial trade with China, the central issue of the controversy was Bethune's politics. Significantly, most of those who defended the government's decision were neither communists nor pro-communist. Their attitude was expressed in a Toronto newspaper's editorial comment: "A few Canadians, not blinded by the fact that he was a Communist, have long been aware that Dr. Bethune was an idealist who practised his ideals, and an exceptionally dedicated and courageous man."

In China, Bethune succeeded in his ambition to serve and be served. His success is his legend.

Source Notes

Many of Bethune's personal letters are in the Bethune File located in the Toronto Room of the Metropolitan Toronto Public Library. References to the material used for the National Film Board production of *Bethune* have been divided into two categories: post-production script (material actually used in the film), and research files (material not used). Information gathered by the author and his research assistants from 1969 to 1973 took the form of letters and taped interviews. The sources of readily accessible information, such as academic records, have not been recorded.

Bethune was an eccentric speller at best, and slight changes in spelling and punctuation have been made in the excerpts from his letters for the sake of clarity.

page	line	A RACE OF PASSIONATE MEN
2	11	Mrs. T.C. McNeice, a longtime resident of Gravenhurt, to author.
2	12	Province of Ontario, Birth Registrations. Bethune celebrated his birthday March 4, despite the officially recorded date.
2	19	Mrs. McNeice.
2	23	Janet M. Cree, a resident of Gravenhurst, to author.

3	27	Janet Cornell to author. The anecdotes concerning Bethune's childhood were related by Mrs. Cornell, Bethune's niece, whose mother was Janet Bethune.
3	33	Letter from Dr. Richard Brown, N.F.B. research files. Bethune often spoke of his early life to Dr. Brown, who worked with him for three months in China.
3	34	Letter from Bethune to Frances Penney, Montreal, January 25, 1929.
3	36	Marion Scott, a close friend of Bethune, to author.
3	39	Harriett Elliston, a friend of Bethune, to author.
4	19	Elwood Robb, a student of Bethune's, to author.
4	21	Allan Smith, a student of Bethune's, to author.
4	29	Elwood Robb.
5	24	Letter from Reverend A. Fitzpatrick to Foreman Robinson, Toronto, October 11, 1911, in the Frontier College Papers, Public Archives of Canada, Ottawa. Frontier College still exists.
5	25	Alfred Fitzpatrick, *The University in Overalls* (Toronto, 1923), Appendix C, p. 160.
5	30	Bethune to Miss McMeeking, the secretary of Frontier College, Whitefish, Ontario, November 12, 1911, Frontier College Papers.
5	36	*Ibid.*
6	2	Bethune to Fitzpatrick, Whitefish, December 31, 1911, Frontier College Papers.
6	7	*Ibid.*
6	16	Bethune to Fitzpatrick, Winnipeg, July 16, 1912, Frontier College Papers.
6	32	Department of National Defence Records. All data concerning his army service is from this source.
7	1	Letter from Dr. E.H. Archibald to Dr. Gabriel Nadeau, April 4, 1941.
7	6	Lillian Smith, a friend of Bethune, to author. There is no record of such a trip in Bethune's army record.
7	37	Dr. C.S. MacDougal, a classmate of Bethune, to author.
7	39	Frederick Campbell Penney, brother of Frances

Penney, to author.

8	7	Dr. W. Pelton Tew to author.
8	12	Dr. MacDougal.
8	26	This information was offered to the author by a colleague of Bethune who wishes to remain anonymous.
8	33	Royal Navy Records. All data concerning his naval service is from this source.
9	11	Annual Report of the Hospital for Sick Children, London, England, 1919, p. 16.
9	25	Dr. Graham Ross, N.F.B. post-production script.
9	28	Letter from Dr. T. Twistington Higgins, N.F.B. research files.
9	34	Dr. Ross to author.
10	4	Janet Cornell.
10	12	Letter from Ruth Patton, N.F.B. research files.
10	17	*Ibid.*
10	26	Ellen Stafford, a resident of Stratford, to author. Miss Stafford obtained this information from a person who does not wish to be identified.
10	29	Mr. S.W. Rust, a patient of Bethune, to author.
10	37	Mary F. Sonnenberg to author.
11	1	Dr. J.G. McDermott, a resident of Ingersoll, to author.
11	7	Dr. Arnold Branch, a colleague of Bethune, to author.
11	15	Data concerning Bethune's air force career was provided by Mr. S.F. Wise, Directorate of History, Canadian Department of National Defence, Ottawa. In a letter to Dean MacCraken of the Detroit College of Medicine and Surgery in January 26, 1925, Bethune included a *curriculum vitae* in which he claimed to have been "Senior Medical Officer and Organizer of the Medical Branch of the Canadian Air Force." A lack of sufficient records in the Canadian Department of National Defence makes it impossible to support or reject Bethune's claim. On his Royal Navy record there is a notation referring to him as "Captain H.N.

Bethune, S.M.O." [Senior Medical Officer? R.J.S.].

11 18 Letter from the Secretary of the West London Hospital, N.F.B. research files.

11 24 Bethune to MacCraken.

11 26 Bethune also worked and studied at two other London Hospitals, the Chelsea Women's Hospital and the Cancer Hospital [Bethune to MacCraken].

11 35 Frederick Penney.

11 38 Mrs. T.L. McColl to author. Mrs. McColl attended school in Edinburgh with Frances and knew her throughout her life.

12 9 *Ibid.*

12 13 The amount was estimated at 10,000 pounds by a near relative who does not wish to be identified.

12 21 Letter from Frances Penney to Ted Allan, co-author of *The Scalpel, The Sword,* December 29, 1942.

12 23 *Ibid.*

12 27 The telegram is in the possession of Janet Cornell.

12 39 Frances to Allan.

13 7 *Ibid.*

13 19 Louis Melzack to author. Mr. Melzack learned this story from Frances when he purchased from her the statue and some of Bethune's books after his death.

13 25 Bethune's *curriculum vitae* stated that he spent two months in 1924 with Dr. Alfred W. Adson, a neurosurgeon at the Mayo Clinic. The Mayo Clinic is unable to confirm this [Clark W. Nelson, Archivist, Mayo Clinic, to author].

THE T.B.'S PROGRESS

14 18 Dr. Edward Kupka, a student and friend of Bethune, to author.

15 9 Bethune to MacCraken. The Detroit College of Medicine and Surgery is now the Faculty of Medicine of Wayne State University.

15 32 Dr. Kupka.

16 3 Dr. H.H. Harris to author.

16	14	Dr. R.C. Rueger, a student of Bethune's, to author.
16	16	Dr. R. Leacock to author.
16	19	Dr. J.G. Christopher, a student of Bethune's, to author.
16	23	Dr. Kupka.
17	12	*Ibid.*
17	29	Frances to Allan.
17	33	Bethune to Frances, Detroit, March 27, 1927.
18	10	Mrs. McColl.
18	12	Frederick Penney.
18	21	Bethune to Frances, Detroit, October 20, 1925.
18	31	Dr. J. Burns Amberson to author.
19	7	Miss Mary Saghi to author.
19	36	Bethune to Frances, undated, but written from Calydor. It would, therefore, have been written between October and December, 1926.
20	27	Bethune to Kupka, Calydor, November 8, 1926.
21	11	All information about the sanatorium can be found in *The Trudeau Sanatorium,* an illustrated booklet describing the nature and costs of treatment, facilities, and conditions of admission.
22	4	George Holt, a friend of Bethune, to author.
22	30	Mrs. Davidson, a student nurse at Trudeau, to author.
22	33	Mrs. W. Steenken, a student nurse at Trudeau, to Mrs. Ruth White, research assistant for the author.
22	36	*Ibid.*
23	9	Dr. John B. Barnwell, N.F.B. post-production script.
23	22	Dr. William S. Schwartz to author.
23	26	Dr. William Steenken to Mrs. White.
23	38	Mrs. Steenken.
24	5	Dr. Barnwell.
24	34	*Ibid.*
25	8	*Ibid.*
25	18	Mrs. Rose Kasner, sister of Dr. Wruble, to Dr. L.L.

Hanawalt, research assistant for the author.

25	24	Letter from Ruth Patton, N.F.B. research files.
25	30	Letter from Bethune to Kupka, Detroit, July 10, 1926.
26	4	Bethune to Frances, Detroit, March 27, 1927.
26	7	File #146805, Records Office of Wayne County, Michigan. Frances had issued a bill of complaint on June 4, 1927. This was followed five days later by a summons served on Bethune by Frances' lawyer, U.S.A. Heggblom. On September 15, 1927, the presentation of an affadavit of the defendant's failure to appear in court resulted in the issuance of an order *pro confesso,* which finds the defendant in default and is an implied admission of guilt.
26	16	Dr. Barnwell.
26	20	*Ibid.*
27	14	A colleague of Bethune, who wishes to remain anonymous, to author.
27	33	*The Trudeau Sanatorium.*
28	11	Dr. Barnwell.
28	21	File #146805
28	23	Dr. Barnwell
29	2	Dr. Earl LeRoy Warren to author.
29	28	This description has been based on Bethune's own commentary on the mural in an article, "The T.B.'s Progress," *The Fluoroscope* (August, 1932), pp. 1 and 10.
30	14	Dr. Barnwell.
30	16	"The T.B.'s Progress," p. 10.
30	40	Trudeau Sanatorium Records.
31	12	"The T.B.'s Progress," p. 1.
31	21	Dan Boice, N.F.B. research files.
31	27	"The T.B.'s Progress," p. 10.
32	10	Dr. Archibald to Dr. Nadeau, December 27, 1940.
32	17	Anonymous doctor to author.
32	24	Dr. David T. Smith to author.
32	29	Bethune, H.N., Smith, D.T., and Wilson, J.L., "The Etiology of Spontaneous Pulmonary Disease in the Albino Rat," *Journal of Bacteriology,* Volume

20 (November, 1930), pp. 361–370.

32   33   Bethune to Kupka, Detroit, July 10, 1926.

SECOND CHANCES

33   13   "Tuberculosis," in *M.D. Medical News Magazine*, 10:8 (August, 1966), p. 181.

33   21   *Ibid.*

34   7   Mitzi Brandtner, a friend of Bethune, to author.

34   9   Henning Sorensen, Bethune's Spanish interpreter, to author.

34   14   P. Harris, "Summary of Tuberculosis Death Rates Per 100,000 Population," Dominion Bureau of Statistics (Ottawa, 1966), as quoted by Dr. F.E. King in *Historical Study of the Voluntary Tuberculosis Community* (Toronto, 1967), p. 20. There were 115.2 deaths per 100,000 population in Quebec in 1925. By 1930, this figure had risen to 118.6.

34   16   M.C. Urquhart and K.A.H. Buckley, *Historical Statistics of Canada* (Toronto, 1965), p. 178. Tuberculosis accounted for the deaths of 2,937 Quebecois in 1925.

34   17   Annual Records, City of Montreal Department of Health, 1925. There were 805 deaths from tuberculosis in Montreal in 1925.

34   19   Dr. Wilder Penfield, "Edward Archibald, 1872–1945," *Canadian Journal of Surgery,* Volume 1 (January, 1958), pp. 167–74. No biography has been written of Archibald, who was the first North American surgeon to employ the technique of thoracoplasty for pulmonary tuberculosis. An excellent outline of his many achievements, including a perceptive description of the man himself, can be found in the above article.

34   33   Letter from Bethune to Frances, Montreal, undated (probably Autumn, 1928).

34   35   All were published in the *Canadian Medical Association Journal* in 1929. For details, see Bibliography.

35   11   Dr. T.J. Quintin, a student of Bethune, to author.

35	24	Norman Bethune, "Some New Thoracic Surgical Instruments," *Canadian Medical Association Journal*, Volume 35 (December, 1936), pp. 656–62.
35	30	Dr. Barnwell.
35	38	"Some New Thoracic Surgical Instruments," p. 659.
36	6	Dr. J.S. Luke to author.
36	16	"Some New Thoracic Surgical Instruments," p. 656.
36	23	Dr. Archibald to Dr. Nadeau, December 27, 1940.
36	26	Dr. Sclater Lewis to author. Dr. Lewis is the author of *Royal Victoria Hospital, 1887–1947* (Montreal: McGill University Press, 1969).
36	29	Bethune to Frances, Montreal, undated (probably Autumn, 1928). The P.P. Cowans Fellowship provided Bethune with a monthly income of $125.00 from July 1, 1928, to March 31, 1931.
36	31	Dr. Arthur Vineberg, a friend of Bethune, to author.
36	35	Dr. C.A. Birch, a colleague of Bethune, to author.
37	9	Beatrice Simon, a friend of Bethune, to author.
37	24	Dr. W.J. MacLeod, N.F.B. research files.
37	37	Dr. Quintin.
38	6	Dr. Birch. Bethune was quoted by the Montreal *Gazette* (April 11, 1934) as saying in an address to the Canadian Progress Club that "the use of the stethoscope without x-ray examination in discovering tuberculosis is nothing more than a farce."
38	22	Dr. Hollis Renton to author.
38	30	Bethune to Frances, Montreal, undated (probably Autumn, 1928).
38	33	*Ibid.*
39	1	Bethune to Frances, Montreal, January 25, 1929.
39	4	Ruth Patton, N.F.B. research files.
39	9	Bethune to Frances, Montreal, undated (probably Autumn, 1928).
39	23	Letter from Dr. John Alexander to Bethune, Ann Arbor, July 1, 1929.

39	34	File #C-144-8-4, Department of Pensions and National Health, National Archives, Ottawa.
40	14	Dr. Ronald Christie to author.
40	19	Dr. H.E. MacDermot to author.
40	29	*Ibid.*
41	9	Dr. Barnwell.
41	17	Louis Huot to author.
41	22	Mitzi Brandtner.
41	37	Dr. D.H. Starkey, a colleague of Bethune, to author.
42	10	Mrs. W.E. Dawson, R.N., a nurse at the Royal Victoria, to author.
42	38	Bethune to Frances, Montreal, undated (probably Autumn, 1928).
43	9	Bethune to Frances, Montreal, January 25, 1929.
43	14	The witnesses were Dr. Graham Ross and Mrs. Norah Wright. Mrs. Wright had attended finishing school with Frances in Paris.
43	29	Bethune to Frances, Great National Park, Arizona, November 30, 1931.
44	19	Bethune to Frances, Mobile, Alabama, December 31, 1931.
44	35	Mrs. Dawson.
45	7	Dr. Christie.
45	19	Dr. Duane Carr to author. Dr. Carr, a thoracic surgeon, was a resident at the University of Michigan at the time.
45	32	Norman Bethune, "A Phrenicectomy Necklace," *American Review of Tuberculosis,* Volume 26 (September, 1932), pp. 319–21.
45	37	Sherman Atwell to author.
46	6	"Some New Thoracic Surgical Instruments," p. 662.
46	9	Dr. Carr.
46	24	Edward Archibald, "Surgery in the Treatment of Pulmonary Tuberculosis," *Canadian Medical Association Journal,* Volume 11, 1921, p. 945.
47	14	Dr. Alan Sampson to author.

47	22	Dr. Walter Mingie to author.
47	26	Dr. Philip Levitsky to author.
48	3	Dr. Vineberg.
48	16	Dr. Hjalmar Larsson, a friend of Bethune, to author.
48	23	Dr. Eugene Osius to author.
48	31	Dorothy Catto, R.N., N.F.B. post-production script.
48	38	Dr. R.H. Overholt to author.
49	2	The description of the conflict between Archibald and Bethune is based on detailed correspondence with Dr. John V.V. Nicholls, a medical student at McGill in 1933. Much of Dr. Nicholls' information was obtained from the late Dr. Stewart Baxter, a Resident in Surgery at the Royal Victoria at the time who knew Archibald well.
49	11	Dr. R. Gordon Townshend to author.
49	22	Dr. Nicholls to author.
49	32	Dr. Archibald to Dr. Nadeau, January 19, 1941.
49	35	Dr. Archibald to Dr. Nadeau, December 27, 1940.
50	3	*Ibid.*
50	8	Louis Huot.
50	22	Dr. V.D. Schaffner, a colleague of Bethune, to author.
50	30	Dr. C.S. Gamble to author.
51	5	Mrs. Dawson.
51	13	Dr. Georges Deshaies, N.F.B. post-production script.
51	19	Henning Sorensen.
51	24	Dr. Luke.
51	30	Dr. Quintin.
52	6	Dr. C.A. McIntosh to author.
52	16	Dr. Aubrey Geddes, N.F.B. post-production script.
52	22	Jean Trenholme, R.N., a nurse at the Royal Victoria, to author.
52	23	Mitzi Brandtner.
52	35	Dr. Christie.
53	7	Louis Huot.

53	13	Irene Kon, a friend of Bethune, to author.
53	21	Dr. Geddes.
53	34	The author of this anecdote does not wish to be identified.
54	10	Dr. Christie.
54	15	Marian Scott.
54	30	Marian Scott, N.F.B. post-production script.
55	8	*Ibid.*
55	26	Louis Huot.
55	34	Dr. Eric Richardson, a friend of Bethune, to author.
56	4	Letter from Bethune to Frances, Calydor, undated (certainly between October and December, 1926).
56	13	George Holt.
56	21	Jean Palardy to author.
56	28	Janet Cornell.
56	31	Marion Scott to author.
56	35	Mitzi Brandtner.
57	5	*Ibid.*
57	13	A.S. Scott to author.

I AM AN ARTIST

58	18	Dr. Luke.
58	20	Minutes of Medical Bureau meeting of Sacré Coeur Hospital, September 24, 1932, p. 79.
59	10	Bethune, probably to Barnwell, N.F.B. post-production script.
59	33	Dr. Georges Cousineau to author.
59	38	*Ibid.*
60	6	Dr. Gérard Rolland, a student of Bethune's, to author.
60	14	Dr. Cousineau
60	26	Dr. L.G. Rigler, a colleague of Bethune, to author.
60	38	Dr. D.T. Smith.
61	37	Dr. Barnwell.
62	7	Lord Brock, Director of the Royal College of Surgeons, London, to author.
62	11	Dr. Edward D. Churchill to author.

62	20	Bethune to Barnwell, Montreal, August 16, 1932.
62	26	Harold Beament to author. Beament, a professional painter and lawyer, advised Bethune on the legal steps necessary to secure the divorce.
62	32	Frances to Allan.
62	37	Louis Huot.
63	7	Bethune to Frances, Montreal, April 12, 1933.
63	11	These women prefer to remain anonymous.
63	39	Frances to Allan.
65	9	Bethune to Frances, Montreal, February 11, 1934.
65	28	Frederick Taylor to author.
66	3	Dr. Geddes.
66	11	Marian Scott, N.F.B. post-production script.
67	31	Bethune to Marian Scott, Madrid, May 5, 1937. In Spain and China Bethune made carbon copies of some of his letters, including this one, which he sent to several friends.
67	37	*Ibid.*
68	2	Marian Scott to author. At least three of Bethune's paintings are extant. "Night Operating Room" is in the private collection of Raymond Boyer of Montreal. A self-portrait is in China, and a third work is in the private collection of Mrs. Aubrey Geddes. A committee under the chairmanship of Dr. Wilder Penfield is in the process of locating "The T.B.'s Progress."
68	20	Marian Scott, N.F.B. post-production script.
68	33	Sylvia Ary, N.F.B. post-production script.
69	7	George Mooney, N.F.B. research files.
69	13	George Holt.
69	15	Marian Scott to author.
69	16	Jean Palardy.
70	13	Norman Bethune, "A Plea for Early Compression," *Canadian Medical Association Journal*, Volume 27 (July, 1932), pp. 36–42.
71	16	These paragraphs are a summary of Bethune's address from the Montreal *Gazette*, April 11, 1934.
71	22	George Mooney. The date is uncertain, although

Mooney suggests that it was late in 1933.

71 32 *Ibid.*

72 5 "Reflections on Return from 'Through the Looking Glass' ", an address delivered to the Montreal Medico-Chirurgical Society, December 20, 1935.

72 11 Dr. Benjamin Potter to author. Dr. Potter accompanied Bethune to Russia.

72 17 "Reflections".

72 23 Jean Palardy.

74 2 "Reflections".

75 7 Memphis *Commercial-Appeal,* February 13, 1936.

75 14 Dr. Carr.

76 24 Minutes of the Montreal Medico-Chirurgical Society, April 17, 1936. Bethune's address was later published as "Take Private Profit Out of Medicine," *Canadian Doctor,* 3:1 (January, 1937), pp. 11–16.

77 10 *Medical Care for the People of Montreal and the Province of Quebec,* pp. 5–6.

78 30 "Take Private Profit . . ."

79 3 Jori Smith, an artist friend of Bethune, to author.

79 15 Bethune to Marian Scott, Montreal, October 8, 1935.

80 2 Stanley Ryerson to author.

81 6 Bethune to Marian Scott, Montreal, October 8, 1935.

81 40 Bethune to Louis Kon, Montreal, October 28, 1935.

82 17 Bethune to Dr. R. Meade, Montreal, February 17, 1936.

82 23 Dr. Carr.

82 40 Gordon McCutcheon to author. McCutcheon, at that time a Party member, met Bethune at a Party meeting.

83 14 Dr. John C. Jones to author.

83 28 Dr. Geddes.

84 27 The woman wishes to remain anonymous.

85 7 Pierre Broué and Emile Témime, *The Revolution and the Civil War in Spain,* translated by Tony White (London: Faber and Faber, 1972), p. 100.

85 22 *Ibid.,* p. 77. The Left won 277 seats from 4,838,499 votes; the Right 132 from 3,996,931; the Centre 32 from 449,320.

87 1 Hugh Thomas, *The Spanish Civil War* (London: Penguin, 1965), p. 219.

87 6 Broué and Témime, p. 183.

88 18 The League Against War and Fascism was a left-wing organization in the United States which lat̲r changed its name to the League for Peace and Democracy.

89 12 Norman Bethune, "Red Moon," Canadian Forum (July, 1937), p. 6.

89 16 Percy Newman to author.

89 21 J.L. Biggar, National Commissioner of the Canadian Red Cross, to Bethune, Toronto, September 18, 1936.

89 25 *The New Commonwealth,* September 26, 1936.

89 30 Graham Spry to author.

90 14 For a complete list of the executive, see Appendix.

90 32 George Mooney, N.F.B. post-production script.

91 6 An article in *The Daily Clarion,* the official Toronto Communist newspaper, stated that Bethune took the following supplies with him: surgical instruments, blood transfusion apparatus, 100,000 units of insulin, 1,000 units each of typhoid and small-pox vaccines, anti-toxin tetanique concentrated, and anti-gangrene serum (*The Daily Clarion,* October 22, 1936).

91 8 New York *Times,* October 26, 1936.

91 15 Thomas, p. 403.

91 30 The words were written by Louis Delaprée, correspondent for *Paris-Soir,* as quoted in Broué and Témime, p. 251.

92 38 Henning Sorensen.

93 19 *Ibid.*

93	28	*Ibid.*
94	6	Bethune to Benjamin Spence, Madrid, December 17, 1936.
94	31	Doctor de la Loma and Dr. Sanz to Fredericka Martin. Miss Martin, a nurse in Spain during the Civil War, is currently writing a history of the American Medical Bureau in Spain.
94	37	Bethune to Spence.
95	7	Telegram from Canadian High Commissioner, London, to Canadian Department of External Affairs, Ottawa, November 27, 1936, in External Affairs File #631–B–36C.
95	14	Memo to Minister of External Affairs from "L.C.C.", a ministerial assistant, November 27, 1936, *ibid.*
95	16	Massey to External Affairs, November 28, 1936, *ibid.*
95	21	Laurent Beaudry, Acting Under Secretary of State for External Affairs, to Spry, October 20, 1936, *ibid.*
95	23	Spry to Beaudry, October 22, 1936, *ibid.*
95	31	"L.C.C." to O.D. Skelton, Under Secretary of External Affairs, November 28, 1936, *ibid.*
96	2	Minister of External Affairs to Massey, November 28, 1936, *ibid.*
96	7	This document is in the N.F.B. research files.
96	9	Bethune to Spence.
96	21	After Franco's triumph, the street was renamed "General Mola" after the Nationalist general who directed the November assault on Madrid and who coined the term "Fifth Column".
96	30	Bethune to Spence.
97	1	Dr. Vicente Goyanes, a member of the Madrid Service, to author. Other members were Dr. Sanz, Dr. Culebras, and Dr. de la Loma.
97	9	*Ibid.*
97	20	Dr. R.S. Saxton, "The Madrid Blood Transfusion Institute," *The Lancet* (September 4, 1937), pp. 606–607. The most common diseases were syphilis

and malaria. Dr. Saxton, a member of the British Ambulance Unit, visited Bethune's service in March, 1937, to study the techniques. Unfortunately, since all records were apparently destroyed, the only specific data, with the exception of infrequent references among Bethune's letters and speeches, is contained in the Saxton article and the notes upon which he based his article. Dr. Saxton has generously supplied the author with a copy of the notes.

97	22	Dr. Saxton. There are four basic blood types under the Moss (I, II, III, IV) or Universal (A, B, AB, O) groupings. Since most Madrileños were either II(A) or IV(O), only these types were taken.
97	24	Henning Sorensen.
97	26	Bethune to Spence.
97	30	Duran Jorda's method was slightly different. Blood in his Barcelona service was stored at 2°–4° C. See Dr. F. Duran Jorda, "The Barcelona Blood Transfusion Service," *The Lancet* (April 1, 1939), pp. 773–775.
97	36	New York *Times,* December 25, 1936.
98	22	Bethune to Spence, Madrid, January 11, 1937.
98	28	Dr. Saxton.
98	38	Bethune to Spence, Madrid, January 11, 1937.
99	11	*Daily Clarion,* January 29, 1937.
99	16	Victor Hoar, *The Mackenzie-Papineau Battalion* (Toronto: Copp Clark, 1969), p. 59.
99	20	Hazen Sise to author.
102	8	Norman Bethune, *The Crime on the Road: Malaga-Almeria* (Madrid: Publicaciones Iberia, 1937).
102	34	*Daily Clarion,* February 17, 1937.
103	4	Henning Sorensen.
103	10	Ted Farah, a Canadian reporter who accompanied Bethune in Paris, to author.
103	18	Thomas, p. 501.
103	27	Henning Sorensen.
103	37	Hazen Sise, N.F.B. post-production script.

104	6	Dr. Albert B. Byrnne, an American doctor working in Spain, to author.
104	9	Herbert Kline to author.
105	4	This letter, probably to Spence, is quoted in the N.F.B. post-production script, but cannot be located.
105	7	Bethune to Marian Scott,. Madrid, February 26, 1937.
105	12	*Daily Clarion,* July 17, 1937.
105	29	The Committee to Aid Spanish Democracy sent $11,656.63 to Spain in 1936 and $17,165.94 in 1937 according to the Auditor's Report, which was accepted at the Committee meeting in Toronto, May 7, 1938.
105	38	Hazen Sise, N.F.B. post-production script.
106	4	Henning Sorensen.
106	12	Fredericka Martin to author.
106	24	Dr. Byrnne.
106	40	Letter from Dr. Muller, N.F.B. research files.
107	4	Louis Huot.
107	7	Herbert Kline.
107	10	Hazen Sise to author.
107	14	Henning Sorensen.
107	18	Montreal *Gazette,* June 8, 1938.
107	19	Hazen Sise to author.

AN EMPTY HOMELAND

108	8	Toronto *Star,* June 15, 1937.
108	17	Montreal *Gazette,* June 19, 1937.
109	8	*Daily Clarion,* September 7, 1937.
109	11	*Ibid.*
109	12	Winnipeg *Free Press,* July 22, 1937.
109	13	*Daily Clarion,* July 26, 1937.
109	18	Bethune to Frances, South Porcupine, Ontario, July 7, 1937.
109	30	George Holt.
110	2	Sault Ste. Marie *Daily Star,* July 14, 1937.

110	5	James Kelleher to author. Mr. Kelleher's father was President of the Rotary Club at the time.
110	20	William Strange, Toronto *Star,* June 15, 1937.
110	24	Winnipeg *Free Press,* July 20, 1937.
110	35	Saskatoon *Star-Phoenix,* August 23, 1937.
111	7	*Northern Daily News* (Kirkland Lake, Ontario), July 6, 1937. MacKenzie King, Prime Minister of Canada, visited Hitler in Germany.
111	14	Professor Elaine Cumming to author.
111	23	Letter from Dr. W. Wilde to Mrs. C.A. Morden, quoted by Mrs. Morden to author.
112	3	Richard Greening to author.
112	11	Dr. Roger Gariepy to author.
112	22	A. Brennan to Editor, *Northern Daily News,* July 13, 1937.
112	37	Dr. Leo Eloesser to author.
113	5	Mrs. Amy Mercer to author. Bethune was the house guest of Professor and Mrs. Mercer.
113	14	Dr. W.J. McLeod.
113	36	Dr. Lewis Fraad to author.
114	5	Miss E. Stirling to author. Miss Stirling chaired the meeting at Salmon Arm.
114	8	The source of this quotation does not wish to be identified.
114	12	Tim Buck to author.
114	32	Dr. Starkey.

HUAN-YING, HUAN-YING

117	32	Dr. Fraad.
117	33	Philip J. Jaffe to author.
118	3	From an unpublished manuscript, *You Can't Buy It Back,* by Jean Ewen, p. 95.
118	12	Dr. Fraad.
118	27	Mrs. Evelyn Kirkpatrick to author.
119	4	*Ibid.*
119	14	Dr. Fraad.
119	22	Bethune to Frances, S.S. Empress of Asia, January 8, 1938.

119	30	Bethune to Marian Scott, S.S. Empress of Asia, January 8, 1938.
120	5	Jean Ewen to author.
120	11	Letter from Bethune to Yenan headquarters, Hu-chia Chuan, May 17, 1938.
120	19	Ewen, p. 103.
120	36	Jean Ewen.
121	23	James Bertram to author.
121	34	The details of their trip are from two sources. The first is an account written by Bethune and published by the Canadian League for Peace and Democracy called *From Hankow to Sian.* It also appeared in some Canadian newspapers in 1938. The second is from Jean Ewen's manuscript. (Abbreviations *H-S* and *YCBB* will be used to designate the sources.)
122	33	Reverend McClure to author.
124	27	*H-S,* p. 1.
125	4	*YCBB,* p. 158.
125	15	*H-S,* p. 7.
125	25	*Loc. cit.*
126	9	*H-S,* p. 8.
126	29	*YCBB,* pp. 154–5.
128	7	*Ibid.,* p. 158.
128	11	*Ibid.,* p. 166.
129	15	Dr. Hatem, a remarkable man who has contributed much to the virtual elimination of venereal disease in China, married a Chinese and has lived in China since 1936.
129	29	*YCBB,* p. 182.
130	40	Dr. Erich Landauer to author.
131	14	Ho Tzu-hsin to author.
131	27	Dr. Landauer.
131	32	Heinrich von Jettmar to author.
132	5	Dr. Ma Hai-te to author.
132	11	Dr. Landauer.

133	13	Ho Tzu-hsin.
134	6	Hsüeh Teng to author.
134	12	Bethune, Sui-te, May 3, 1938. This letter, one of the carbon-copied "Letters to Canada", is in the N.F.B. research files and has no addressee.
134	31	Ho Tzu-hsin.
135	17	Letter from Bethune to Yenan headquarters, May 17, 1938.
136	12	*Ibid.*
136	26	Bethune proposed a monthly operating budget of $1250.
137	1	Letter from Bethune to Dr. Robert S.K. Lim, Wu-t'ai Mountains, July 19, 1938.
137	16	Bethune to Yenan.
137	35	Tung Yüeh-ch'ien, *Throughout the Green Mountains*, p. 1. Tung was Bethune's interpreter. *Throughout the Green Mountains* is one of ten essays written about Bethune by Chinese who knew him and collected in one volume, *The Great Internationalist Soldier Bethune* (Peking: China Youth Publishing House, 1965).
139	18	Bethune to Lim.
139	22	Letter from Bethune to Ma, Sung-yen K'ou, July 19, 1938.
139	25	*Ibid.*
140	5	Bethune to Elsie Siff, Wu-t'ai Mountains, July 19, 1938.
140	13	Letter from Bethune to Yenan headquarters, Hu-chia Chuan, May 22, 1938.
140	21	Bethune, *Analysis of Work from May 1, 1938, to July 20, 1938, of the Canadian-American Mobile Medical Unit.* Copies were sent to General Nieh, Mao Tse-tung, and the American League for Peace and Democracy.
141	32	An Chih-lan, head nurse at Ho-chien Hsien, to author.
141	36	Ho Tzu-hsin.

142   2   Dr. Brown. N.F.B. post-production script.

142   19   *Ibid.*

142   30   Nieh Jung-chen, from a "Report at General Headquarters of the Eighth Route Army," October 13, 1944.

143   5   Dr. Chang Yeh-shang, one of Bethune's assistants, to author.

143   31   Letter from Bethune to General Nieh, Sung-yen K'ou, August 13, 1938.

144   6   Chou Kuang-t'ien, a nurse at Sung-yen K'ou, to author.

144   17   Bethune to Yenan Military Council, August 11, 1938.

145   10   N.F.B. research files.

146   10   Bethune's *November Report of the Canadian-American Mobile Medical Unit to General Nieh,* Yang-chia Chuang, December 7, 1938.

147   13   *Ibid.*

147   31   Hsüeh Teng.

147   33   No documentation could be located for the date of this appointment. Letters as late as November were signed "Norman Bethune, Surgeon, Canadian-American Mobile Medical Unit" or simply "Norman Bethune, M.D." The first time the title "Medical Advisor" appears among the letters is in a "Letter to Canada" dated January 10, 1939. The appointment was probably made in the early autumn of 1938.

148   9   Lang Lin to author.

148   23   George Mooney, Diary, April 2, 1946. Mr. Mooney was a guest of General Nieh in China when Mooney served with the United Nations Relief and Rehabilitation Administration.

149   8   Bethune's *Speech at the Opening of the Model Hospital at Sung-yen K'ou,* September 15, 1938.

149   39   Bethune to Ma, Yang-chia Chuang, December 8, 1938.

150   18   Bethune, "Letter to Canada," Yang-chia Chuang, January 10, 1939.

150	33	Dr. Yeh Ching-shan, a doctor who worked with Bethune, to author.
151	22	Bethune, Diary, March 1, 1939. This is one of four diary extracts published in the Chinese biography of Bethune, *Bethune's Path*, by Wei Ai (Hong Kong: Wen-chiao Publishing Co., 1970).
152	10	An Chih-lan.
152	19	*Ibid.*
152	28	Ho Tzu-hsin.
152	35	Dr. Yeh Ching-shan.
153	3	An Chih-lan.
153	9	Feng Ch'ing-chung, a medical assistant to Bethune, to author.
153	17	An Chih-lan.
153	24	Dr. Chang Yeh-shang.
154	3	Bethune's "Report to Committees in New York, Hong Kong and London," Shen-pei, July 1, 1939.
154	9	Dr. Chang Yeh-shang.
154	24	July Report.
154	32	Dr. Ch'en Chi-yüan, a medical assistant to Bethune, to author.
155	2	July Report.
155	14	*Ibid.*
156	3	Bethune, "Monthly Report of Canadian-American Mobile Operating Unit," August 1, 1939.
156	18	None of these books is known to be extant, and the Chinese themselves are eager to find them.
157	11	Bethune to Louis Davidson, on the border of north-western Hopei, August 15, 1939.
157	22	Bethune to general headquarters of Chin-Ch'a-Chi Military Region, August 16, 1939.
157	27	Bethune to Davidson.
158	5	Lang Lin.
158	33	Bethune to Barnwell, August 15, 1939. This was the same letter Bethune sent to Davidson with the exception of his remarks concerning the China Aid Council.
159	2	Dr. Chang Yeh-shang.

159   21   Dr. Yeh Ching-shan.

160   21   *Ibid.*

160   31   An Chih-lan.

163   40   Dr. Ma.

164   5   Nieh Jung-chen to author.

164   18   The other two are *The Foolish Old Man Who Removed the Mountains* and *Serve the People. In Memory of Norman Bethune* is reprinted in the Appendix.

164   35   The telegram was sent to the China Aid Council in New York.

165   18   Minutes of the 1943 annual convention of the Canadian Labour Congress.

165   22   Ted Allan and Sydney Gordon, *The Scalpel, The Sword* (Toronto: McClelland and Stewart, 1952).

165   38   The film distribution is no longer restricted.

166   22   In a letter to the author, March 8, 1972, Peter H. Bennett, Assistant Director (Historic Sites), National and Historic Parks Branch, Department of Indian and Northern Affairs wrote: 'The subject (of naming Bethune a Canadian of National Historic significance) had been discussed at several previous meetings and at the meeting in October 1971, a conclusion was reached. By that time copious documentation had been assembled and the Board was in possession of a medical assessment obtained through the Medical Research Council to view his achievements in the context of the history of medicine in Canada. It was recommended that Dr. Bethune's career was not of national historic importance.' "

167   12   Toronto *Star*, August 18, 1972.

167   23   Toronto *Globe and Mail*, August 19, 1972.

Appendix A

A BRIEF GENEALOGY OF THE BETHUNES

Normandy was the home of the first known Bethunes, some of whom left France in the eleventh century and went to Scotland during the reign of Malcolm III. Aggressive, intelligent and strong-willed, the Bethunes of Scotland were eminent in the clergy. Among them were David, Cardinal Beaton (1494–1546), and James Beaton, Archbishop of Glasgow and Primate of Scotland. Several members of the family were physicians on the Isle of Skye.

The Bethunes were noted for their courage and independence. After the Battle of Culloden and the imposition of English law and religion on the Scots, John Bethune (1751–1815), a minister of the dissenting Church of Scotland, left his native Isle of Skye and settled in America. Although in Scotland he had opposed English domination, he remained loyal to the Crown during the War of Independence and was imprisoned by the Americans. Following his release, he went to Montreal and built Saint Gabriel Street Church, the first Presbyterian church in Canada.

Three of Reverend Bethune's six sons were conservative businessmen and two were clerics. John (1791–1872), an Anglican priest, was Rector of Montreal for fifty-four years, as well as

Dean of Montreal and Principal of McGill University. Alexander Neil (1800–1879) was educated by John Strachan, the first Bishop of Toronto, and succeeded Strachan on his death in 1867. His son Charles James Stewart (1838–1932) was also ordained in the Church of England and became the first Head Master of Trinity College School in Port Hope, Ontario, a boys' school which he made famous throughout North America during his thirty-year term.

Angus Bethune (1783–1815) rejected the staid life of his five brothers. Rugged and individualistic, he went into the Canadian wilderness to trap for furs. By 1814 he had raised himself to the position of Partner in the North West Company. When his company merged seven years later with the Hudson's Bay Company, he was appointed a Chief Factor. His son Norman (1822–1892) was born at Moose Factory on Hudson Bay. Angus had made enough money from the fur trade to send Norman to Toronto for an education, which included private tutoring from his uncle Alexander Neil. After graduation from Upper Canada College and King's College in Toronto he went to Britain to study medicine. In 1850 he was granted his medical degree from Edinburgh University.

Norman inherited his father's independent spirit. Although he had been educated by his Anglican uncle, he later joined the Presbyterian Church, possibly as the result of a conflict with the Anglican authorities at Trinity University in Toronto. He and five medical colleagues founded Trinity Medical School in 1850, but the school, which originally had no religious requirements for entry, was closed in its sixth year when Dean Bethune and his entire faculty resigned in protest against a new university regulation that barred non-Anglicans. Restless, talented, and ambitious like his father, Norman travelled during the next fifteen years. He practised surgery in Edinburgh, where he married Janet Nicolson in 1856, and crossed the Atlantic working as a ship's surgeon. His diaries reveal considerable literary skill, and he was a talented amateur painter. In 1871, Trinity Medical School re-opened with a non-sectarian admissions policy, and he returned to Toronto to teach at Trinity and practise medicine. He died there in 1892, survived by his son Malcolm Nicolson (1857–1932), the father of Norman Bethune (1890–1939).

Malcolm Goodwin, Norman's brother, died in 1944. One nephew, Douglas, and four nieces survive Norman: They are Mrs. Janet Cornell, Mrs. Ruth Neily, Mrs. Joan Lindley, and Mrs. Helen Lowes.

Appendix B

EXECUTIVE OF THE COMMITTEE TO AID SPANISH DEMOCRACY

Officers

Honorary Chairman:
Rev. Dr. Salem G. Bland
Chairman:
Rev. Benjamin H. Spence
Vice-Chairmen:
Graham Spry, Dr. Rose Henderson,
Tim Buck, A.A. McLeod
Secretary:
E.E. Wollon
Financial Secretary:
Norman Freed
Treasurer:
Bruce Robinson

The Executive comprised the Officers and the following: Stewart Smith, D. Nesbitt, J.M. Connor, Mrs. Annie Buller, Fred Collins, E.M. Aplin, Harold Potter, Mrs. Elizabeth Morton, David Goldstick, S.B. Watson.
Also included on the Executive were the chairmen of the representative committees from various provinces: Maritimes—D.W. Morrison; Quebec—J. Cupello; Manitoba—Hon. E.J. McMurray, K.C.; Saskatchewan—George Williams; Alberta—Harold Gerry; British Columbia—A.M. Stephen.

Appendix C

IN MEMORY OF NORMAN BETHUNE

Comrade Norman Bethune, a member of the Communist Party of Canada, was around fifty when he was sent by the Communist Parties of Canada and the United States to China; he made light of travelling thousands of miles to help us in our War of Resistance Against Japan. He arrived in Yenan in the spring of last year, went to work in the Wutai Mountains, and to our great sorrow died a martyr at his post. What kind of spirit is this that makes a foreigner selflessly adopt the cause of the Chinese people's liberation as his own? It is the spirit of internationalism, the spirit of communism, from which every Chinese Communist must learn. Leninism teaches that the world revolution can only succeed if the proletariat of the capitalist countries supports the struggle for liberation of the colonial and semi-colonial peoples and if the proletariat of the colonies and semi-colonies supports that of the proletariat of the capitalist countries. Comrade Bethune put this Leninist line into practice. We Chinese Communists must also follow this line in our practice. We must unite with the proletariat of all the capitalist countries, with the proletariat of Japan, Britain, the United States, Germany, Italy and all other capitalist countries, for this is the only way to overthrow imperialism, to liberate our nation and people and to liberate the other nations and peoples of the world. This is our internationalism, the internationalism with which we oppose both narrow nationalism and narrow patriotism.

Comrade Bethune's spirit, his utter devotion to others without any thought of self, was shown in his great sense of responsibility in his work and his great warm-heartedness towards all comrades and the people. Every Communist must learn from him. There are not a few people who are irresponsible in their work, preferring the light and shirking the heavy, passing the burdensome tasks on to others and choosing the easy ones for themselves. At every turn they think of themselves before others. When they make some small contribution, they swell with pride and brag about it for fear that others will not know. They feel no warmth towards comrades and the people but are cold, indifferent and apathetic. In truth such people are not Communists, or at least cannot be counted as devoted Communists. No one who returned from the front failed to express admiration for Bethune whenever his name was mentioned, and none remained unmoved by his spirit. In the Shansi-Chahar-Hopei border area, no soldier or civilian was unmoved who had been treated by Dr. Bethune or had seen how he worked. Every Communist must learn this true communist spirit from Comrade Bethune.

Comrade Bethune was a doctor, the art of healing was his profession and he was constantly perfecting his skill, which stood very high in the Eighth Route Army's medical service. His example is an excellent lesson for those people who wish to change their work the moment they see something different and for those who despise technical work as of no consequence or as promising no future.

Comrade Bethune and I met only once. Afterwards he wrote me many letters. But I was busy, and I wrote him only one letter and do not even know if he ever received it. I am deeply grieved over his death. Now we are all commemorating him, which shows how profoundly his spirit inspires everyone. We must all learn the spirit of absolute selflessness from him. With this spirit everyone can be very useful to the people. A man's ability may be great or small, but if he has this spirit, he is already noble-minded and pure, a man of moral integrity and above vulgar interests, a man who is of value to the people.

Mao Tse-tung
Yenan, December 21, 1939

Further Acknowledgements

The following supplied information from hospitals:

Mary Weil, Royal Victoria Hospital, Montreal
The Director, Sacré Coeur Hospital, Montreal
Grace Hamlyn, Royal Edward Chest Hospital, Montreal
Judith McGibbons, Reddy Memorial Hospital, Montreal
Barbara Johnson, Harper Hospital, Detroit
B. Garton, Royal Free Hospital, London
W.J. Taylor, West London Hospital, London
T.A. Ramsay, North East Metropolitan Regional Hospital
  Board, London
A.E. Whitsworth, Queen Charlotte's and Chelsea Hospitals,
  London
I. Kent, Royal Marsden Hospital, London
P.W. Dixon, Hospital for Sick Children, London
D.W. Tindall, Queen Mary's Hospital for the East End,
  London
P.A. Lake, Hammersmith and St. Mark's Hospital, London

Data was obtained from the following educational institutions:

Jesse Ketchum Public School, Toronto
Owen Sound Collegiate and Vocational School
University of Toronto
Royal College of Surgeons, Edinburgh

198

The following provided documentation from libraries and other institutions:

Raymond Chu, Library, Department of East Asian Studies, University of Toronto
Nancy Young, Library, College of Education, University of Toronto
The Staff, Academy of Medicine, Toronto
Hugh MacMillan, Province of Ontario Archives, Toronto
Robert J. Taylor, Dominion Archives, Ottawa
Dr. J.D. Wallace, Canadian Medical Association, Ottawa
G.W. Hillborn, Archives, Department of External Affairs, Ottawa
S.F. Wise, Directorate of History, Department of National Defence, Ottawa
G.E. Logan, Records Division, Department of National Health and Welfare, Ottawa
Margaret Farmer, Medical Library, McGill University
Susan Biggs, Osler Library, McGill University
Sandra Guillaume, Archives, McGill University
Rohan Butler, British Foreign Office
Miss G.M. Thorp, Ministry of Defence, London
W.A. MacMillan, Churchill Livingstone Co., London
Clark Nelson, Archives, Mayo Clinic, Rochester
Victor Berch, Special Collections Library, Brandeis University
Jack Delehant, Trudeau Institute, Saranac Lake

The following were of invaluable assistance to me in my collection of information in the People's Republic of China:

Huang Hua, Ambassador of the People's Republic of China to the United Nations
The Chinese Medical Association
The Chinese People's Association for Friendship and Understanding with Foreign Countries
The Staff of the Norman Bethune International Peace Hospital, Shih-chia Chuang
Dr. Ma Hai-Te
Nieh Jung-chen, Vice-Premier, People's Republic of China

I wish also to thank the following:

Dr. A.L. Abel, I. Abramowitz, Dr. F.D. Ackman, Dr. P. Adolph, Ted Allan, Julio Alvarez del Vayo, Paul Andrew, Ted Aplin, Robert Ayre, Thelma Ayre, Kate Bader, Dr. J. Bain, T.J. Baleanter, Mary Balfour, Dr. H. Ballon, Sonia Bank, Helen Barbour, Harold Beament, Dr. Harold Beeson, Dr. Paul Beeson, Dr. Edward Bensley, Dr. P. Beregoff-Gillow, Dr. G. Bernath, Dr. M. Berne, Syd Birdsey, Dr. J.D. Bisgard, Raymond Boyer, Dr. Benjamin Brock, Fred Brodie, Earl Browder, Dr. Lyla Brown, Elisabeth Browne, Dr. J.L.S. Browne, Mrs. T.C. Browne, Tim Buck, Dr. C.B. Buffam, Ted Burke, Dorothy Cameron, Helen Campbell, Sam Carr, Eveline Carsman, Dr. H.R. Carstens, Mary Cash, Dr. Paul Chapman, John Christensen, Dr. J.G. Christopher, Dr. Muir Clapper, Paraskeva Clark, Dr. Owen Clarke, John Clout, Dr. R.D. Coddington, Mrs. Sam Colle, Dr. W. Condon, Dr. Gordon Copping, Dr. Charles Cossage, Muriel Coy, Jack Cranmer-Byng, Dr. Leon Crome, Barnett Danson, Marjorie Darrach, Dr. J.A. Davidson, Dr. H.L. Dawson, Dr. J.J. Day, William Dennison, Dr. Orville Denstedt, Mrs. Georges Deshaies, Dr. J. Dinan, Dr. W.J. Downs, Dr. René Dumont, Jeannie Eady, Lucy Easlick, Dr. K.A.C. Elliott, Dr. Leo Eloesser, Professor Shinkichi Eto, Dr. Gerald Evans, Bruce Ewen, Roy Faibish, Dr. I.S. Falk, Dr. W.B. Faulkner, Beatrice Ferneyhough, Mrs. G. Fidlar, Dr. Walter Fischer, Murray Fischer, Eileen Flanagan, R.N., L.C. Fletcher, Sr., M. Fleury, R.N., Stuart Forbes, Ronald Freeman, Dr. A.G. Frost, Dr. Godfrey Gale, Dr. C.S. Gamble, Dr. Roger Gariepy, H. Gaston, R.N., Mrs. Aubrey Geddes, Martha Gelhorn, Carol George, Mary Goldie, Dr. Vicente Goyanes, Dr. Greenberg, Dr. Robert Greenblatt, Richard Greening, Dr. J. Guasch, Dr. Francisco Guerra, C.L.B. Hall, Dr. John Hamilton, Catherine Hammond, Dr. Joaquin d'Harcourt, Dr. Fred Harper, Georgetta Harper, Dr. H.H. Harris, Dr. M.S. Harris, Professor Robin Harris, Allan Harrison, Dr. Alex Tudor Hart, Dr. Jerome Head, U.S.A. Heggblom, Professor Keiichi Hirano, Victor Hoar, Dr. C.L. Hodge, Dr. F.W. Holcomb, Dr. G.A. Holland, Michael Horn, Dr. Perry Hough, J.E. Houghton, Dr. John Howlett, Dr. A. Hunt, Leslie Hunt, Dr. H.J. Irwin, Mary Carter Isbell, Dr. H. von Jettmar, Dr. A.F. Jones, Dr. H.I. Jones, Walter Judd, Geza Karpathi (Charles Korvin), William Kashtan, Roy Keffer, John Kemeney, Robert Kenny, Dr. Frederick Kergin, W. King, Ethel Klein-

stein, Irene Kon, Dr. Alberto Ladron de Guevara, James Larkin,
Dr. Hjalmar Larsson, Dr. R.C. Leacock, Dr. Leon Leahy, Nor-
man Lee, Dr. Rachmael Levine, Harvey Levinson, Dr. Sclater
Lewis, Professor Paul Lin, Dorothy Livesay, Dr. A.L. Lockwood,
Dr. Valentin de la Loma, Dr. J.G. Lynch, Anne MacDermott,
Janet MacKay, R.N., Hugh MacLennan, Dr. Maurice Malins,
Mary Marinich, Herbert Matthews, Dr. G.B. Maughan, Dr. W.D.
Maycock, Dr. J.E. McArthur, Dr. F.C. McCrimmon, Marjorie
McEnaney, Tom McEwen, Marguerite McIntyre, Marjorie
McKenzie, Dr. Francis McNaughton, Amy Mercer, Dr. J.B.
Mickie, Dr. W. Mingie, M. Mokry, Mrs. T. Mooney, Dr. R.
Moore, G.A. Morden, R.N., Nigel Morgan, Anna Taft Mulda-
vin, Dr. Gordon Murray, Dr. R.G. Nelson, Dr. J.V. Nicholls,
Dr. Myron Notkin. Dr. W.H. Oatway Jr., Dr. Alton Ochsner,
Dr. R. Palmer, Libby Park, Dr. J. Parnley, Steve Pascos, Dr.
F. Griffith Pearson, C.O.H. Pease, Dr. Carleton Peirce, Dr. Wil-
der Penfield, Dr. W. Pike, Dr. Juan Planelles, E.R. Powell, Dr.
José Puche, Harold Redman, Mrs. C.E. Reeves, Dr. Hollis Ren-
ton, Grace Reynolds, Mac Reynolds, Dr. J.V. Riches, Dr. Leo
Rigler, T.W. Ritchie, Lea Roback, David Robinson, Nora Rodd,
Fred Rose, Dr. Charles Rosen, Robin Ross, Dr. T.E. Roy, Dr.
Joseph Rubinstein, Dr. R.C. Rueger, Amy Russell, Stanley Rust,
Dr. Charles Ryan, Dr. D.A. Sampson, Charles Sanders, Dr.
Reginald Saxton, Dr. V.D. Schaffner, Dr. Charles Schnee, Dr.
Rose Schneider, Sylvia Schwartz, Dr. W. Schwartz, Professor
F.R. Scott, Dr. John Scott, Dr. F.C. Scott-Moncrief, Dr. J.B.
Scriver, Celia Seborer, Dr. Segal, Dr. H. Shapiro, Robert Shaw,
Cecil Shell, Gerry Simmons, Dr. George Simpson, Edgar Snow,
Helen Foster Snow, Dr. Saul Solomon, Dr. Leslie Soper, Ellen
Stafford, Professor Joseph Starobin, Miss E. Stirling, Dr. John
Streider, Dr. Earnest Struthers, Muni Taub, Dr. G.D. Taylor,
Dr. Andrew Thomson, Dr. Gordon Townshend, Jean Tren-
holme, R.N., Dr. J. Trueta, Alex del Turbine, Louise Vezina,
Dr. André Sanz Vilaplana, Dr. Roger Violette, Elizabeth Wal-
lace, Joe Wallace, Dr. D.R. Webster, Dr. Paul Weil, Saul Well-
man, H. Whitaker, R.N., Mrs. Ruth White, Dr. DeWitt Wilcox,
R.B. Williams, Dr. Julius Lane Wilson, Dr. R.A. Wilson, Mrs.
W. Woodruff, Norah Wright, Mary Young, Dr. W.J.F. Young,
Michael Boland.

Bibliography

Bethune's Writings

Four excerpts from Bethune's diary can be found in the Chinese biography of Bethune by Wei Ai, *Bethune's Path* (Hong Kong: Wen-chiao Publishing Co., 1970).
The Crime on the Road: Malaga to Almeria. Madrid: Publicaciones Iberia, 1937. (descriptive essay)
"The Dud." Toronto *Clarion*, July 8, 1939. (short story)
"Encounter." (unpublished short story in the possession of Marion Scott)
From Hankow to Sian. Toronto: Canadian League for Peace and Democracy, 1938. (travel account)
"Red Moon." *Canadian Forum,* Vol. 17 (July, 1937). (poem)
"Wounds," in Horn, J.S., *Away With All Pests* (London: Hamlyn and Co., 1969). (descriptive essay)

MEDICAL ARTICLES
"Some new instruments for injection of lipiodol: oil-guns and combined cannula and mirror," *Canadian Medical Association Journal (CMAJ),* Vol. 20 (March, 1929), pp. 286–7.
"Note on bacteriological diagnosis of spirochaetosis of lungs," *CMAJ*, Vol. 20 (April, 1929), pp. 265–8.
"New combined aspirator and artificial pneumothorax apparatus," *CMAJ*, Vol. 20 (June, 1929), p. 663.

"Technique of bronchography for general practitioner," *CMAJ*, Vol. 21 (December, 1929), pp. 662–7.

(with) Smith, D.T. and Wilson, J.L. "Etiology of spontaneous pulmonary disease in the albino rat," *Journal of Bacteriology*, Vol. 20 (November, 1930), pp. 361–70.

"Plea for early compression in pulmonary tuberculosis," *CMAJ*, Vol. 27 (July, 1932), pp. 36–42.

"Phrenicectomy necklace," *American Review of Tuberculosis*, Vol. 26 (September, 1932), pp. 319–21.

"Cotton-seed oil in progressively obliterative artificial pneumothorax," *American Review of Tuberculosis*, Vol. 26 (December, 1932), pp. 763–70.

"Silver clip method of preventing haemorrhage while severing interpleural adhesions, with note on transillumination," *Journal of Thoracic Surgery (JTS)*, Vol. 2 (February, 1933), pp. 302–306.

(with) Moffatt, W. "Experimental pulmonary aspergillosis with aspergillus niger; superimposition of this fungus on primary pulmonary tuberculosis," *JTS*, Vol. 3 (October, 1933), pp. 86–98.

"Case of chronic thoracic empyema treated with maggots," *CMAJ*, Vol. 32 (March, 1935), pp. 301–302.

"Pleural poudrage; new technique for deliberate production of pleural adhesions as preliminary to lobectomy," *JTS*, Vol. 4 (February, 1935), pp. 251–61.

"Maggot and allantoin therapy in tuberculosis and non-tuberculous suppurative lesions of lung and pleura: report of eight cases," *JTS*, Vol. 5 (February, 1936), pp. 322–9.

"Some new thoracic surgical instruments," *CMAJ*, Vol. 35 (December, 1936), pp. 656–62.

Secondary Sources

BOOKS

Allan, Ted, and Gordon, Sydney. *The Scalpel, The Sword*. Toronto: McClelland and Stewart, 1952.

Anon. ed. *The Great Internationalist Soldier Bethune*. Peking: China Youth Publishing House, 1965.

Kovich, Jean Ewen. *You Can't Buy It Back*. (unpublished manuscript)

Wei Ai. *Bethune's Path*. Hong Kong: Wen-chiao Publishing Co., 1970.

204

ARTICLES

Farah, Ted. "Canada's Blood Trust in Spain," *Canadian Magazine,* August, 1937, pp. 22–23.

Fish, F.H. "Dr. Norman Bethune," *Calgary Associate Clinic Historical Bulletin,* 10:4 (February, 1946) pp. 151–9.

Hirano, Keiichi. "Jerome Martell and Norman Bethune—a note on Hugh MacLennan's *The Watch That Ends the Night,*" paper read at the 39th General Meeting of the English Literary Society of Japan, May 27–8, 1967.

Larsson, B.H. "In Memoriam: Norman Bethune, M.D.," *Detroit Medical News,* 44:38 (May, 1953).

MacDermott, Anne. "The Only Canadian the Chinese Ever Heard Of," *Maclean's,* May, 1962, pp. 18–19, 62–4.

Nadeau, G.A. "A T.B.'s Progress," *Bulletin of the History of Medicine,* Vol. 8 (October, 1940).

OBITUARIES

Eloesser, Leo, *Journal of Thoracic Surgery,* Vol. 9 (April, 1940), pp. 460–62.

Fisher, L., *American Review of Tuberculosis,* Vol. 41 (June, 1940), pp. 819–21.

Index